CAN

WHY WE'RE STILL DYING TO KNOW THE TRUTH

PHILLIP DAY

 Credence Publications

Cancer - Why We're Still Dying to Know the Truth

Copyright © 1999
Phillip Day

The right of Phillip Day to be identified as the Author of the
Work has been asserted by him in accordance with the
Copyright, Designs and Patents Act 1988.

Printing History

First Edition	April 1999
Second Edition	January 2000
Third Edition	January 2001

First published in 1999
by Credence Publications

Manufactured in the United Kingdom by

Credence Publications
PO Box 3
TONBRIDGE
Kent TN12 9ZY
UK
www.credence.org

3rd Ed. VS

Table of Contents

Introduction

Hello. My name is Phillip Day, and I am very pleased to meet you. You're reading this book either because you became curious and bought it, or maybe you are a cancer sufferer who received it anonymously from a well-intentioned friend or relative. Some people buy copies and pass them out to their families because they feel the information contained within these pages can quite literally save a loved one's life. Actually it doesn't really matter how you ended up with my book in your hands, only that you have!

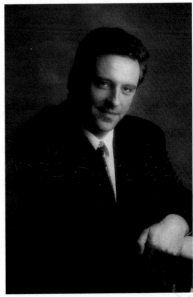

What follows, I believe, is quite simply the greatest medical story of the 20th century – the search for and discovery of the real answer to cancer. The information you are about to read was first broadcast with the publishing of G Edward Griffin's book, *World Without Cancer* in 1974. For reasons we will discuss, Griffin and the cancer researchers for whom he spoke surprisingly experienced repeated, ferocious attacks over their revelations by orthodox medicine. Health authorities and government agencies spared no effort to bury this astounding information with outright lies, false accusations and deceit. But time, integrity and the incredible testimonies of the healed bear witness indeed that the information Griffin reported was correct as scientific, empirical and demonstrable truth. Yet the lies and disinformation about cancer continue to this day. And so does the battle to prevent the real treatments from becoming known.

There is no family in the western world that has not suffered cancer. Who is not familiar with this king scourge of diseases that seems to defy all attempts of modern science to defeat it? Many members of my family have died of this most debilitating of conditions over the years. We were compelled to watch as our loved ones were transformed from happy, carefree and active people into ravaged humanity with no will left to live. We are surely not alone. Every reader has his or her own story to tell about those cancer deaths which left their family mourning, overwhelmed by a sense of uselessness and hopelessness that still none of our specialists and super technology were yet capable of writing the final epitaph of cancer and burying it forever.

Well, the good news is here! This book is a celebration of a profound hope in the war against cancer and other degenerative diseases and is the result of many years' research into the cancer industry. In fact, as we will see, the true story of cancer mostly typifies a battle, not only against the condition of cancer itself, but also against the politics, economics and attitudes which have sprung up like strangling weeds around one of the greatest health killers of the 20th century.

Before we begin, let's first get the disclaimer out of the way. Please allow me to describe who I am and what this book is and what it isn't. I am not a doctor, a medical practitioner, an oncologist or healthcare specialist, I am a reporter/researcher and have been working in this field for over twelve years. While I am not qualified to issue medical advice of any kind, I am certainly qualified to collate and pass on medical information and report statements put out by medical researchers and practitioners. My speciality is uncovering suppressed truths that have been withheld from the public, usually to serve the ends of some covert agenda. Neither is this book just a wilful treatise on conspiracy, although, as we will discover, conspiracy has ever been in the mind of man, especially with those who stand to make a vast fortune at somebody else's expense.

This book does not seek to gainsay the advice and recommendations of qualified medical personnel and their institutions in individual situations. Clinical cancer is of course a serious condition and professional healthcare specialists should always be consulted, whether the intended treatment is to be chemically or nutritionally based.

The facts presented in this book are intended for informational and educational purposes only and must in no way be construed as medical advice. The purpose of this book is to allow the reader to exercise a valuable right – the right to informed consent; in other words, the right to make a decision on cancer prevention techniques or choosing a cancer therapy based on as much evidence as is currently available. At the present time, certainly in the realm of cancer, this right is being deliberately denied you.

You are about to read a catalogue of the facts surrounding the historic search for the answer to cancer and the people involved in this plight. This book is a reporting of their words and of suppressed information in relation to the struggle to make the treatment and prevention of cancer known to all. Ultimately it must be left to you the reader to ponder on what you are about to learn and make your own determination on how best to proceed from this point forward.

It is sad that a disclaimer such as this is necessary when thousands are dying each day through lack of knowledge. But, as we shall see, there are those who are passionate about you not learning what you are about to read in the coming pages, and then there are always those who will abuse and misapply any information to their own or someone else's harm. The story of cancer isn't simply about finding a magic bullet and then announcing the cure to the cheers of all. To believe so would be to demonstrate an unrealistic naiveté about the medical/chemical industries and the commercial dynamos that drive them.

Are people healing themselves of cancer? Yes... TEN THOUSAND TIMES YES!! No, we are not talking about a few isolated cases. You can discover as you read how ordinary men and women, sent home to die by the doctors and specialists they trusted, resolved to survive against the odds simply by going back to basics and studying the facts of their condition for themselves.

The information in this book will surprise and anger those who have lost loved ones to cancer - and well it should. The current state of affairs is simply unacceptable to the many who have followed the progress of the doctors and medical researchers who press on with the true work regardless of the intimidation that still dogs them. These valiant professionals are well on their way to spread the wonderful news worldwide that, for decades now, it has been over for cancer; that cancer need not be the Terminator, even for those already diagnosed with it.

If there is, concerning cancer, a sadder truth than the millions who have needlessly perished through lack of knowledge, it is the lies, duplicity and shame practised within the highly profitable medical and chemical industries which are proving rather more indestructible than the disease itself. And so, let us begin.

Can We Ever Beat Cancer?

The American Cancer Society states that this year around 590,000 Americans will die from cancer. From a disease which killed approximately 1 in 750 of us at the turn of the 1900s, cancer has grown over the years to become a major health disaster due to claim at least one in every two to three of us. In a few short years, experts predict, cancer will surpass heart attack/disease as the No.1 killer of humankind in the western world. If this exponential rise is allowed to continue unchecked well into the next century, the cancer incidence is predicted to approach 100%.

Breast cancer serves as a poignant yardstick. This type of malignancy is now the leading cause of death in women between the ages of 35 and 54. In 1971, a woman's lifetime risk of contracting breast cancer was 1 in 14[1]. Today it is 1 in 8. *Rachel's Environment and Health Weekly*, No. 571 reports: *"More American women have died of breast cancer in the past two decades than all the Americans killed in World War 1, World War 2, the Korean War and Vietnam War combined."*

Cancer certainly seems to be unstoppable and is believed to be so by the majority of the public today. Yes, we see recoveries, but these appear to be the exception rather than the rule. There plainly doesn't seem to be any consistency in who makes it and who doesn't. Yet, as we will discover, the reality is that there are civilisations and peoples existing today *who do not suffer from cancer and indeed cannot record one victim of the disease in their culture.*

Can we beat cancer? Yes. It's already done. The knowledge to conquer cancer was understood many decades ago but the facts never made it into the public domain until relatively recently. With the development of the Internet, the information you are reading is now available to all who care to research it, and yet amazingly, the truth is still suppressed, lies disseminated, people hounded and

---

[1] **Epstein, Dr Samuel S & David Steinman** The Breast Cancer Prevention Program, Macmillan, USA, 1997 ISBN 0025361929

jailed in order to protect a voracious and highly profitable corporate agenda.

The Politics of Cancer

The information you are about to read is not supported, endorsed or accredited by any official government body or medical institution. Rather, today's practitioners of establishment medicine have come to label the information contained in this book 'quackery' and 'delusion', even though official, well-documented studies and some of the world's top cancer specialists support the efficacy of the treatments we will be discussing in the following pages. Ironically, we will discover as we proceed that the charges of 'quackery' and 'delusion' are now being increasingly levelled back at the cancer industry itself over the use of unproven, toxic drugs and radiation treatments which have a well-documented record of ending life rather than prolonging it.

The politics of cancer as they stand today are simple. Cancer drugs are a multi-billion-dollar industry to the pharmaceutical companies which make their money patenting and selling chemical drug treatments to the public. There are powerful corporate interests extremely keen to keep it this way. The *proven* preventatives and treatments for cancer, on the other hand, *cannot be patented*. Why? Because the techniques are preventative in nature (and therefore not patentable) and the active ingredients are available to anybody no further away than your local supermarket, waiting for you to eat them!

Clearly if ever it became common knowledge that there was a simple answer to cancer, the monopoly enjoyed by these pharmaceutical conglomerates would evaporate very quickly - and of course the huge profits that go along with it. Thus, as we will see, extraordinary legal measures have been taken by these corporations, government agencies and international cartels to ensure that their gravy train is kept firmly on the rails.

The book *World Without Cancer* was the whistleblower for which many had yearned who already sensed an underlying corporate cancer agenda at work[2]. Before we examine parts of his book, a word about the author himself. Mr Griffin, whom I had the privilege of meeting briefly in the summer of 1995 in Westlake Village, California, is a writer and documentary film producer with many titles to his credit. He is listed in *Who's Who* in America and is renowned for his talent for researching difficult topics and reporting them to the public in simple, easy-to-understand language. He is a graduate of the University of Michigan, majoring in speech and communications and is a recipient of the Telly Award for excellence in television production. He is founder of the Cancer Cure Foundation and has served on the board of directors of the National Health Federation and the International Association of Cancer Victims and Friends.

Edward Griffin took upon himself the task of collating a wide spectrum of data concerning the war on cancer – and not only a war on the disease itself, but a war between two opposing parties: the medical establishment and a small group of its medical researchers and doctors who fervently believed they had found the answer to the disease. Griffin was originally alerted when his friend Dr John Richardson made it known that he had stumbled across a revolutionary new way of looking at cancer and the means to treat it.

Using a safe and natural substance, the basis of which was freely available in any grocer's store, Richardson had been successfully treating terminally ill cancer patients when combining this substance with detoxification and nutrition techniques, much to the outrage of fellow members of the medical profession. The American Medical Association, the American Cancer Society and indeed members of the hospital where he practised turned on Dr Richardson, labelling him 'a quack' and putting pressure on him to abandon his unorthodox research. Upon questioning the reasons behind such inexplicable opposition to news for which the world was desperately waiting, Griffin began a three-year research project destined to uncover the most unsavoury facts about the

[2] **Griffin, G Edward** *World Without Cancer*, American Media, 1996 ISBN 0912986190 (Available through Credence at www.credence.org)

medical/chemical industries and the professionals in whom we have all come to trust.

Griffin writes: *"In the years prior to World War II, there came into existence an international drug cartel, centered in Germany, that dominated the entire world's chemical and drug industries. It had spread its operations to ninety-three countries and was a powerful economic and political force in all countries. It was known as I G Farben."*

I G Farben was later to be the mainstay behind much of Hitler's chemical production during the war years, manufacturing products which included high explosive, battlefield poison gas and the infamous Zyklon-B, the deadly agent used in the extermination camps of the Nazis. Neither was I G Farben happy to run its empire through intermediaries. Among those administering the death camp Auschwitz-Birkenau were I G Farben personnel, the ring-leaders of whom were later tried for their crimes at Nuremburg. Prior to the war in 1928 however, American industrial monopolist John D Rockefeller had established a combine between his American-based international empire and I G Farben, producing the largest and most powerful drug cartel the world had ever known. This organisation exists today, under various names and structures, and plays a major role in both the science and politics of cancer therapy.

The Rockefellers knew well the science of creating a need and then filling it to massive profit. New substances began to be licensed proprietarily as 'drugs' and approved by the Rockefeller-sponsored American Medical Association and Food & Drug Administration, with doctors and specialists trained in their dispensation and use through Rockefeller-financed institutions.

Griffin reports: *"Abraham Flexner, author of the famous Flexner Report of 1910, led the crusade for upgrading the medical schools of America, all the while he was in the employ of Andrew Carnegie and John D Rockefeller, who had set up gigantic tax-exempt foundations for that purpose. The end result was that all medical schools became heavily oriented towards drugs and drug research, for it was through the increased sale of drugs that the donors realized a profit on their donations.*

A brief backward glance at the total landscape will help us appreciate more fully the present extent of cartel influence, not only in the FDA (United States Food & Drug Administration) but at all levels of the federal government. The list of men who are or were in key positions within the Rockefeller group reads like a 'Who's Who' in government[3]."

Rockefeller money almost single-handedly transformed medicine from the old-fashioned barber's shop practices into the modern, well-organised allopathic[4] industry we recognise today. JD's organisational abilities were legendary in the projects to which he turned his hand and impressive fortune. Ironically JD's father William had peddled quack remedies off the back of his wagon in the mid-1800s. But his son was to have altogether more grandiose designs. Largely through JD's efforts, doctors underwent the metamorphosis from poorly paid wagon-quacks to sophisticated, well-educated and highly paid luminaries, trained in Rockefeller drug-lore in the new colleges funded and built by Rockefeller and Carnegie. Foundations were formed; chemical research financed. The 20th century began with obvious medical promise of great deeds to come.

This apparent beneficial turn for mankind's healthcare however was to have some unfortunate repercussions in the realm of monopoly abuses. 'Alternative' and unpatentable treatments not sanctioned by the new medical infrastructure were routinely pilloried and given little press coverage. Gradually the public came to accept that the new drugs had become the only perceived and plausible players in the war against the dreaded cancer[5].

---

[3] Griffin, G Edward, ibid.

[4] **allopathy** – orthodox medical practice, treatment of diseases by drugs.

[5] **Mullins, Eustace** *Murder by Injection*, Iconoclast Books, Ketchum, ID USA

Does 'Conventional' Treatment Work?

And so the chief medical quest throughout the first half of the 20th century was to conquer cancer and other illnesses with chemicals or drugs. Millions of dollars were ploughed into the pharmaceutical multi-nationals in an effort to research effective treatments for the many different types of cancer, for it had become rapidly evident that a 'magic bullet' cure would not be forthcoming overnight. Millions of laboratory animals were slaughtered, and indeed continue to be killed around the world in the search for a cancer drug cure.

As John Rockefeller progressed with his monopolisation of the American pharmaceutical industry and the inauguration of the American Medical Association and Food & Drug Administration, the harshest experiments were conducted at New York's Memorial Hospital, the victims of the debilitating disease subjected to the most heinous treatments with Marie Curie's radium and other desperate 'remedies'. Very few survived the medicine (including Marie Curie), let alone the cancer itself[6]. Things have changed little, although the experiments continue worldwide. Today, the conspicuous failure of chemotherapy (toxic drugs) and radiotherapy (the use of x-rays) to halt the major cancers has become evident even to the medical practitioners who prescribe them.

The first matter for us to consider is whether or not traditional, drug-based medicine has had any quantitative success in treating or regressing cancer. As either someone who has been diagnosed with cancer or one who is interested in 'just not getting it', the reader may certainly find this important to establish. We read newspaper articles almost daily on medicine's heroic 'victories' or 'breakthroughs' with drugs, but here we have to ask the uncomfortable question: Does modern medicine really have the answer to cancer or are we just being snowed?

---

[6] Mullins, Eustace, ibid.

Christian Brothers writes as follows: *"Scientific American featured a recent cover story entitled: "The War on Cancer -- It's Being Lost." In it, eminent epidemiologist John C. Bailar III, MD, PhD, Chairman of the Department of Epidemiology and Biostatistics at McGill University cited the relentless increase in cancer deaths in the face of growing use of toxic chemotherapy. He concluded that scientists must look in new directions if they are ever to make progress against this unremitting killer[7].*

Adding its voice, the prestigious British medical journal The Lancet, *decrying the failure of conventional therapy to stop the rise in breast cancer deaths, noted the discrepancy between public perception and reality. "If one were to believe all the media hype, the triumphalism of the* [medical] *profession in published research, and the almost weekly miracle breakthroughs trumpeted by the cancer charities, one might be surprised that women are dying at all from this cancer," it observed. Noting that conventional therapies - chemotherapy, radiation and surgery - had been pushed to their limits with dismal results, the editorial called on researchers to "challenge dogma and redirect research efforts along more fruitful lines[8]."*

John Cairns, professor of microbiology at Harvard University, recorded in his scathing 1985 critique in *Scientific American*: *"Aside from certain rare cancers, it is not possible to detect any sudden changes in the death rates for any of the major cancers that could be credited to chemotherapy. Whether any of the common cancers can be cured by chemotherapy has yet to be established."*

Making the point that chemotherapy is *not* curative, and actually has very little effect on the major cancers, Dr Martin F Shapiro stated in the *Los Angeles Times* that *"...while some oncologists inform their patients of the lack of evidence that treatments work... others may well be misled by scientific papers*

---

[7] See also: "Progress Against Cancer?" *New England Journal of Medicine*, May 8, 1986, p. 1231

[8] Christian Brothers, http://www.christianbrothers.com.

that express unwarranted optimism about chemotherapy. Still others respond to an economic incentive. <u>Physicians can earn much more money running active chemotherapy practices than they can providing solace and relief... to dying patients and their families[9]</u>."

These testimonials have been made by 'conventional' doctors and medical research specialists who have reputations at stake. These statements would be shocking enough on their own if they were the only dissenting voices in today's $7 billion chemotherapy industry. They are not. If one does the homework, one finds statements from doctors and oncologists who are repeatedly coming out in desperation against traditional cancer treatments for one simple and straightforward reason – they don't see them working. We will examine further testimonies as we proceed.

The cancer institution is huge business today employing multitudes and earning billions worldwide. It is a fact that today there are more people making a living from cancer than are dying from it. History has shown that some corporations are prepared to do and say almost anything to protect their lucrative incomes, as we have seen with the tobacco industry. Has this happened with cancer?

A blistering indictment of Cancer Inc. was delivered by Dr Samuel Epstein at a press conference in Washington DC on 4th February 1992. The statement was co-authored by former directors of three US federal agencies and endorsed by 64 leading national experts in cancer prevention, public health, and preventative medicine[10]. The indictment read, in part:

"We express concerns that the generously funded cancer establishment, the National Cancer Institute (NCI), the American Cancer Society (ACS) and some twenty comprehensive cancer centers, have misled and confused the public and Congress by repeated claims that we are winning the war against cancer....

---

[9] *Los Angeles Times*, 9th January 1991

[10] A list of these is held with Credence Publications.

Cancer now strikes one in three and kills one in four Americans, with over 500,000 deaths last year. Over the last decade, some 5 million Americans died of cancer and there is growing evidence that a substantial proportion of these deaths was avoidable....

Furthermore, the cancer establishment and major pharmaceutical companies have repeatedly made extravagant and unfounded claims for dramatic advances in the treatment and "cure" of cancer. Such claims are generally based on an initial reduction in tumor size ("tumor response") rather than on prolongation of survival, let alone on the quality of life, which is often devastated by highly toxic treatments[11]."

Cancer provides an income for millions of people. One is tempted to ask why on earth, from a business standpoint, anyone would ever want to cure it. This question has occurred to many honest physicians who have become thoroughly uneasy over the years with the party line and the nature of the treatments they are obliged to foster.

Alan C Nixon, PhD, erstwhile President of the American Chemical Society, declares that *"...as a chemist trained to interpret data, it is incomprehensible to me that physicians can ignore the clear evidence that chemotherapy does much, much more harm than good."*

Oncologist Albert Braverman MD told the world in 1991 that *"...no disseminated neoplasm (cancer) incurable in 1975 is curable today... Many medical oncologists recommend chemotherapy for virtually any tumor, <u>with a hopefulness undiscouraged by almost invariable failure.</u>"*

Christian Brothers: *"In 1986, McGill Cancer Center scientists sent a questionnaire to 118 doctors who treated non-small-cell lung cancer. More than 3/4 of them recruited patients and carried out trials of toxic drugs for lung cancer. They were asked to imagine*

---

[11] A copy of this report may be downloaded from www.preventcancer.com

that they themselves had cancer, and were asked which of six current trials they themselves would choose. 64 of the 79 respondents would not consent to be in a trial containing cisplatin, a common chemotherapy drug. Fifty-eight found all the trials unacceptable. Their reason? The ineffectiveness of chemotherapy and its unacceptable degree of toxicity[12]".

Dr Ralph Moss was the Assistant Director of Public Affairs at probably America's most famous cancer research institution, Memorial Sloan Kettering in Manhattan. He states: *"In the end, there is no proof that chemotherapy in the vast majority of cases actually extends life, and this is the GREAT LIE about chemotherapy, that somehow there is a correlation between shrinking a tumor and extending the life of a patient[13]."*

Christian Brothers further reports: *"There are more and more reports by establishment oncologists doubting the value of chemotherapy, even to the point of rejecting it outright. One of these, cancer biostatistician Dr Ulrich Abel, of Heidelberg, Germany, issued a monograph entitled 'Chemotherapy of Advanced Epithelial Cancer' in 1990[14]. Epithelial cancers comprise the most common forms of adenocarcinoma: lung, breast, prostate, colon, etc. After ten years as a statistician in clinical oncology, Abel became increasingly uneasy. "A sober and unprejudiced analysis of the literature," he wrote, "has rarely revealed any therapeutic success by the regimens in question in treating advanced epithelial cancer."*

While chemotherapy is being used more and more extensively, more than a million people die worldwide of these cancers annually - and a majority have received some form of chemotherapy before dying. Abel further concluded, after polling hundreds of cancer doctors, "The personal view of many oncologists seems to be in striking contrast to communications intended for the public." Abel cited studies that have shown "...that many oncologists would not

---

[12] Christian Brothers, ibid.
[13] Live on the Laurie Lee Radio Show, 1994
[14] *Healing Journal,* No. 1-2, Vol.7 of the Gerson Institute

take chemotherapy themselves if they had cancer[15]. *Even though toxic drugs often do effect a response, a partial or complete shrinkage of the tumor, this reduction does not prolong expected survival," Abel finds. "Sometimes, in fact, the cancer returns more aggressively than before, since the chemo fosters the growth of resistant cell lines." Besides, the chemo has severely damaged the body's own defenses, the immune system and often the kidneys as well as the liver*[16].*"*

Dr Abel displays the results of chemotherapy in patients with various types of cancers as the improvement of survival rates compared to untreated patients. This table shows:

Colorectal cancer:	no evidence survival is improved.
Gastric cancer:	no clear evidence.
Pancreatic cancer:	study completely negative. *Longer survival in control (untreated) group.*
Bladder:	no clinical trial done.
Breast cancer:	no direct evidence that chemotherapy prolongs survival; its use is "ethically questionable." (That is particularly newsworthy, since all breast cancer patients, before or after surgery, are given chemotherapy drugs.)
Ovarian cancer:	no direct evidence.
Cervical/uterine:	no improved survival.
Head and neck:	no survival benefit but occasional shrinkage of tumours.

Christian Brothers again: *"In the Wall Street Journal, 17*[th] *November 1994, in a front-page article describing political pressure exerted on insurance companies to pay for bone marrow transplants in advanced breast cancer, experts give a totally negative report on this approach. The procedure, called ABMT (Autologous Bone Marrow Transplant) involves temporarily*

---

[15] *The Cancer Chronicles,* December 1990
[16] Christian Brothers, ibid.

removing some of the patient's bone marrow, applying a potentially lethal dose of chemotherapy, then returning the marrow to the patient's body. The cost of this procedure is in excess of $100,000[17]."

Professor Charles Mathe, French cancer specialist, makes this astonishing declaration: *"If I contracted cancer, I would never go to a standard cancer treatment centre. Cancer victims who live far from such centres have a chance*[18]*."*

Walter Last, writing in *The Ecologist*, reports: *"After analysing cancer survival statistics for several decades, Dr Hardin Jones, Professor at the University of California, concluded in 1975 that "...patients are as well, or better off untreated." Jones' disturbing assessment has never been refuted. What's more, three studies by other researchers have upheld his theory*[19]*."*

Paul Winter writes: *"It is not likely that any doctor knowingly suppresses a cancer cure to protect their business or career. But every doctor has his or her own ideas about the best treatment based on what they have learned. The pharmaceutical companies however have an extremely strong influence over what medical doctors are taught. Doctors are too busy to dig into the statistics of cancer treatments, they assume that what they are taught at school or what is demonstrated in the pages of briefing journals is the best treatment. They cannot afford to suspect that these treatments are only the best for the pharmaceutical companies that influence their 'institutions of higher learning'.*[20]*"*

That hospitals and clinics could, in themselves, be dangerous to our health is rarely considered by the average layman whose respect for doctors and medicine borders on worship. Figures

---

[17] Christian Brothers, ibid.
[18] **Mathe, Prof. George** "Scientific Medicine Stymied", *Medicines Nouvelles* (Paris) 1989
[19] *The Ecologist,* Vol 28, No. 2, March/April 1998, p. 120
[20] **Winter, Paul** *The Cancell Home Page,* http://www.best.com/handpen/Cancell/cancell.htm

released in 1998 and published in *Environment and Health News* make sobering reading:

"Australians may want to think twice before their next trip to the clinic. The chances of dying in hospital, or suffering some injury while there, stand at around 16% in Australia. Half this risk is due to doctor or hospital error – which means that 8% of hospital patients are accidentally killed or injured by the staff[21]."

In January 1993, Ralph Nader's American consumer watchdog organisation released the results of a three-year study of American hospitals. The bottom line of the report's conclusion was that 300,000 Americans were killed every year in hospitals alone as a result of medical negligence. Nader took the unprecedented step and used the word 'killed'. He was referring to wrong prescriptions, errant and incompetent medical procedures, and so on. 300,000 Americans every year were simply... killed.

In July of 2000, the Journal of the American Medical Association was to confirm the figure at a conservative 250,000[22]. This figure is equivalent to over five times the number of active American service personnel who were killed in the entire Vietnam War (dodging bullets and bombs) *perishing EVERY YEAR at the hands of their doctors.* Even at the time of writing, two doctors have hit the headlines in England for allegedly causing the death of 12-year-old cancer victim Ritchie William through medical negligence. This case is the tip of the iceberg for allopathic medicine, whose surgical cancer procedures, together with toxic, radioactive chemicals with strongly questionable efficacy, cause thousands misery, mutilation and death on a daily basis.

Britain's *Daily Mail* reported in its front page article on 27th December 1999: *"At least 230 Britons die each day because the National Health Service is the sick man of Europe.... The deaths, from cancer, lung disease and heart disease amount to an astonishing 84,000 a year and stem from poor treatment in*

---

[21] *Environment and Health News*, Vol. 3, Jan 1998
[22] *Journal of the American Medical Association*, Vol. 284 26th July 2000

Britain's Third World wards compared with the best available in the rest of Europe."

The mortality rate quoted by the *Daily Mail* incredibly approaches the average number of British civilian and military personnel who were being killed in combat during one of the past century's most devastating conflicts - World War 2. The study, commissioned by the Bow Group think tank and authored by researcher Chris Philp, also stated that these numbers may be on the low side because the study *"...did not look at all cancers and other diseases which claim lives within the NHS every day."*

Drs. John Diamond and Lee Cowden give this scathing summary of their experience of 'Cancer Inc': *"To the cancer establishment, a cancer patient is a profit center. The actual clinical and scientific evidence does not support the claims of the cancer industry. Conventional cancer treatments are in place as the law of the land because they pay, not heal, the best. Decades of the politics-of-cancer-as-usual have kept you from knowing this, and will continue to do so unless you wake up to their reality[23]."*

Why is it that the scandals concerning cancer treatment remain muted? Mostly because doctors have not yet fully realised the fraudulence of the cancer industry and the greed which drives it. Paul Winter explains: *"Even if you have the best doctors, their information about alternative cancer treatments is probably incorrect. Doctors are so busy that they must rely on summaries of medical research or testing. These summaries are usually prepared by institutions that oppose alternative treatments.... If you carefully research other alternative cancer treatments you will find the same type of disinformation. How and why this happens is thoroughly explained in the book,* The Cancer Industry *by Dr Ralph Moss[24]."*

---

[23] **Diamond, Dr John and Dr Lee Cowden** *Alternative Medicine: The Definitive Guide to Cancer*, Future Medicine Publishing, Inc, 21-1/2 Main St, Tiburon, CA 94920 pp.643-647 (800) 333-HEAL. Excerpted at whale.to/politics/politics.html
[24] **Moss, Ralph W** *The Cancer Industry: The Classic Exposé on the Cancer Establishment*, Equinox Press, 1995 ISBN 1881025098

W Deutscher makes the following colossal statement that equally applies to our malaise of medical peer adoration and collective national error regarding traditional cancer therapies:

"We concentrate on consistency without much concern of what it is we are being consistent about, or whether we are consistently right or wrong. As a consequence, we have been learning a great deal about how to follow an incorrect cause with the maximum of precision[25]."

---

[25] **Deutscher, W** *Social Problems*, University of Manchester Institute of Science and Technology course hand-out

The Good News

But into the misery of cancer came a ray of light. Researcher Joe Vialls explains: *"During 1950 after many years of research, a dedicated biochemist by the name of Ernst T. Krebs, Jr., isolated a new vitamin that he numbered B17 and called 'laetrile'. As the years rolled by, thousands became convinced that Krebs had finally found the complete control for all cancers, a conviction that even more people share today. Back in 1950, Ernst Krebs could have had little idea of the hornet's nest he was about to stir up. The pharmaceutical multinationals, unable to patent or claim exclusive rights to the vitamin, launched a propaganda attack of unprecedented viciousness against B17, despite the fact that hard proof of its efficiency in controlling all forms of cancer surrounds us in overwhelming abundance[26]."*

Ernst Theodor Krebs Jr. was born in Carson City, Nevada. He attended medical college in Philadelphia from 1938-41 and received his AB degree from the University of Illinois in 1942. He was a graduate student at the University of California Berkeley (UCB) from 1943-45 and researched in pharmacy from 1942-45. Krebs and his father are also credited with pioneering the medical applications for Vitamin B15 or pangamic acid, a nutrient largely embargoed by the medical establishment. During the pre-war years, Krebs concentrated his studies on the knowledge and use of enzymes, including bromelain, chymotrypsin, trypsin and papain, in the treatment of cancer. Both Krebs and his father are widely recognised today as the pioneers of Vitamin B17, otherwise known as amygdalin or laetrile, in its role in the treatment of cancer.

'Nitrilosides' are natural foods rich in Vitamin B17. This vitamin is characterised by a large group of water-soluble, essentially non-toxic, sugary compounds found in over 800 plants, many of which are edible. One of the most common sources of B17 is found in plentiful supply within the kernels (seeds) of many non-citrus fruits, such as cherries, nectarines, peaches, plums and apples[27].

---

[26] **Vialls, Joe** *Laetrile: Another Suppression Story*, www.livelinks.com/sumeria
[27] *Economic Botany* (30:395-407, 1963)

However it is within the seed of the humble apricot that the highest concentrations of B17 can be found, up to 2 to 2.5 percent by weight in most varieties.

Krebs went to work on his new discovery and interfaced what he had learned about B17 with the research of a doctor living thirty years before. In Griffin's *World Without Cancer,* the author explains Krebs' research in the light of the trophoblastic theory of cancer proposed by Professor John Beard of Edinburgh University. Beard was an embryologist and one of the first specialists to study the enigmatic embryonic stem cells that are contained within our bodies.

These cells are arrested at the pre-embryonic stage and have not yet gone on to develop into the cell structure of the body parts they repair and replenish on an on-going basis. Beard's research revealed that stem cells in pregnancy (trophoblasts) do not vary in any discernible way from highly malignant cancer cells. The trophoblast cells are necessary for the growth of the new embryo, but after the 56th day of pregnancy, the baby's new pancreas begins emitting the chymotrypsin enzyme and the trophoblast is killed off from that point forward.

Griffin writes: *"The trophoblast in pregnancy indeed does exhibit all the classical characteristics of cancer. It spreads and multiplies rapidly as it eats its way into the uterus wall preparing a place where the embryo can attach itself for maternal protection and nourishment[28]."*

Joe Vialls continues: *"The trophoblast is formed in a chain reaction by another cell* [stem cell] *that Griffin simplifies down to the 'total life' cell, which has the total capacity to evolve into any organ or tissue, or a complete embryo. When the total life cell is triggered into producing trophoblast by contact with the hormone estrogen, present in both males and females, one of two different things happens. In the case of pregnancy the result is conventional development of a placenta and umbilical cord. If the trophoblast is*

---

[28] Griffin, G Edward *World Without Cancer,* ibid.

triggered as part of a healing process however, the result is cancer or, as Edward Griffin cautions: "To be more accurate, we should say it is cancer if the healing process is not terminated upon completion of its task[29]."

A trophoblast cell (a stem cell triggered by estrogen) produces quantities of chorionic gonadotrophin (hCG) which can be detected in urine with a simple test that is 92% accurate in all cases. In regard to a positive test result, Griffin notes: *"If the patient is a woman, she is either pregnant or has cancer. If he is a man, cancer can be the only cause[30]."* Yet the medical industry, in full possession and knowledge of this information and associated tests, still insists on recommending dangerous biopsy operations to detect cancerous growths, the biopsies themselves sometimes contributing to the spread of cancer cells through the body when cuts in the tumours are made.

Beard's conclusions back at the turn of the 1900s were astonishing and have never been overturned. In his Unitarian or Trophoblastic Thesis of Cancer, Beard stated that cancer was simply a healing process that wasn't terminating, due to inadequate supplies of pancreatic enzymes. Later it would be found that diets rich in animal proteins depleted these vital supplies of pancreatic enzyme agents in the body, leaving heavy meat/animal-protein eaters vulnerable to cancer.

Krebs was putting together another intriguing piece of the cancer puzzle. The biochemist was aware of a number of cultures on Earth who just did not suffer cancer, heart disease, diabetes and other degenerative conditions, but who lived to ages in many cases exceeding 120 years. He recognised that these peoples lived in non-toxic environments and consumed foods that were minerally abundant, containing nitrilosides rich in hydrocyanic acid[31]. Krebs later isolated hydrocyanic acid from apricot seeds and prepared it in a crystalline form for consumption. He named the

---

[29] Vialls, Joe, ibid.

[30] Griffin, G Edward *World Without Cancer,* ibid.

[31] For a list of forty of the most common foods containing Vitamin B17, please refer to the Appendix…

nutrient laetrile. Later, under advice of Dr Dean Burk, co-founder of the National Cancer Institute, the substance was to receive the controversial designation – Vitamin B17.

Krebs' studies showed that when a human or animal system ingests sufficient amounts of laetrile (or its natural form, hydrocyanic acid), this substance becomes selectively toxic to trophoblast or cancer cells. Analysis revealed a remarkable profile for the reaction that subsequently followed. Hydrocyanic acid is stable, chemically inert and non-toxic when taken as food or as a refined pharmaceutical in appropriate quantities (laetrile/amygdalin). However Krebs discovered the compound reactes to the enzyme beta-glucosidase, located in huge quantities at the site of cancerous tumours, but not to any degree anywhere else in the body. In this reaction, beta-glucosidase manufactures two potent poisons at the cancer cell site: hydrogen cyanide and benzaldehyde (an analgesic/painkiller), stabilised with two molecules of glucose. These two poisons, produced in minute quantities, combine synergistically to produce a super-poison many times more deadly than either substance in isolation. The cancer cell meets its chemical death at the hands of Vitamin B17's selective toxicity.

Krebs was aware that indigenous peoples consuming vast quantities of hydrocyanic acid were not experiencing any harmful side-effects from this reaction – on the contrary, their lives were characterised by abundant good health and extreme longevity. Krebs wanted to know what happened to the excess Vitamin B17 that was being produced and not consumed in the killing of malignant trophoblast.

He discovered that all healthy cells (NOT trophoblast/cancer cells) contain another enzyme, rhodanese, which acts as the control agent. Rhodanese is present within the body in inverse proportions to beta-glucosidase. In other words, it is common throughout the body *yet not at cancerous locations.* If B17 comes into contact with healthy cells, rhodanese detoxifies the cyanide and oxidises the benzaldehyde, which of course means that B17 is accurately targeted *only at cancerous locations and not at healthy tissue.* The two by-products of the rhodanese reaction, thiocyanate and benzoic acid, are actually beneficial in nourishing healthy cells - the thiocyanate taken into the liver to form the metabolic pool for the production of Vitamin B12 (cyanocobalomin). An excess of these by-products is expelled in normal fashion from the body via the urine.

Krebs published his report on laetrile.

And the real cancer war began.

What is Cancer?

There are certain things we know about cancer. We are aware that cancer is caused by environmental toxins – but how? We know that cancer is a chronic disease - that is, it will persist and not clear up by itself without intervention - but is there a way to combat ALL cancers? The fact that cancer is a chronic disease tells us our immune system cannot combat cancer by itself – an important point we will examine a little further on.

But there is another fact about cancer that is not so widely recognised by the general public. Cancer is a metabolic disease. It seems to be connected in some way to diet.

In 1936, the startling Document #264 was issued by the United States Senate. It stated in part:

"Our physical well-being is more directly dependent upon minerals we take into our systems than upon calories or vitamins, or upon precise proportions of starch, protein or carbohydrates we consume... Do you know that most of us today are suffering from certain dangerous diet deficiencies which cannot be remedied until depleted soils from which our food comes are brought into proper mineral balance?

The alarming fact is that foods (fruits, vegetables and grains), now being raised on millions of acres of land that no longer contain enough of certain minerals, are starving us - no matter how much of them we eat. No man of today can eat enough fruits and vegetables to supply his system with the minerals he requires for perfect health because his stomach isn't big enough to hold them."

Farmers are paid for bushel and ton yields of crops per acre. No farmer is paid for putting minerals and nutrients back into the soil beyond those, like NPK, that directly affect the bounty of his harvest. In fact, so severely depleted of nutrients have our farm soils become, that in many areas today seeds won't germinate without the presence of fertilizer. Consequently minerals vital to the

28

maintenance of our health have been largely absent from our food chain, and a whole range of metabolic deficiency diseases have arisen to strike us as a result. Mineral deficiency in our farm soils was an extremely pressing issue for the US Senate back in the 1930s! Do you think the situation has got any better?

Nothing was done.

A controversial, but little-known fact is that more than a few of the nutritional deficiency diseases mankind suffers from today have been cured in livestock for decades. The reason this has been done is because farming livestock is an economic necessity, and so solving recurring health problems with commercial livestock was given top priority by veterinarians in order to safeguard the economic viability of food production. I grew up on a farm and know firsthand that animal feed is fortified with vitamins and minerals.

Put another way, if we treated our farm animals with the same healthcare philosophy with which we treat ourselves today (cure, not prevention), our steaks would cost $240 in the local supermarket and our woolly sweaters would need to be paid for on finance. Conversely, if we were to treat ourselves with the same nutritional and prevention common sense with which we care for our commercial livestock, we wouldn't need $200 a month health plans, Blue Cross, Blue Shield and the creaking British National Health Service. We would simply be giving our bodies the correct raw materials they need to maintain optimum health and avoiding the minefields. Why is the current state of affairs in healthcare the way it is? Because, like it or not, curing sickness is BIG BUSINESS, while promoting the prevention ethic isn't.

The sad reality is, our present populations are falling sick with nutritional deficiency diseases which could easily be avoided by supplementing the vitamins and minerals that have gone missing in the food chain and amending our worthless diets. Yet we have now been conditioned to such a degree that most of us view modern medicine and its doctors, not nutrition, as the vital safeguards for our future health and well-being. And oh, how we are prepared to pay for the privilege.

Another distressing fact is that medicine very often misses the plot when it comes to solving some of mankind's most serious diseases. The 'virus hunters', who dominate the grant-hungry medical research communities worldwide, see a microbe behind every serious disease. Billions have been spent chasing down non-existent viruses for scurvy, cancer, AIDS, Legionnaires', SMON, pellagra and many other ailments, with a criminal disregard for the obvious evidence that suggests completely non-viral and far more simple causes for these illnesses[32]. Ernst Krebs remarks:

"There are many chronic or metabolic diseases that have challenged medicine. Many of these diseases have already been conquered. What proved to be their solution? By solution we mean prevention and cure. What really cures really prevents. Let us think of some of these diseases that have found total prevention and hence cure.

At one time, the metabolic disease known as scurvy killed hundreds of thousands of people, sometimes entire populations. This disease found total prevention and cure in the ascorbic acid or Vitamin C component of fruits and vegetables. Similarly, the once fatal diseases so aptly called pernicious anemia, pellagra, beriberi, countless neuropathies, and the like, found complete cure and prevention in specific dietary factors, that is, <u>essential nutrients in an adequate diet</u>[33]."

Concerning cancer, Dr Harold W Manner[34] writes as follows: *"In recent years a significant reassessment of the nature and*

---

[32] **Day, Phillip & Steven Ransom** *World Without AIDS*, Credence Publications, 2000 ISBN 0953501256

[33] **Krebs, Ernst T** *Journal of Applied Nutrition*, Vol. 22, Numbers 3 & 4, 1970

[34] Dr Harold Manner was chairman of the biology department at Loyola University in Chicago during the 1970s. Because of institutional harassment over his decision to treat cancer patients with laetrile, he moved to Tijuana, Mexico where he ran the Manner Clinic, successfully treating thousands of US cancer patients from 1982 until his death in 1992.

causes of cancer has taken place. Cancer was formerly believed to be a localized disease, characterized by a lesion, usually in the form of a growth, which appeared at some specific part of the body. This localized lesion was thought to be the result of activity produced by an invading virus, carcinogenic agent or some form of trauma such as a blow.

Today, there is a growing conviction among researchers and physicians that cancer is a complex disease that is the end result of a disturbed metabolism (body chemistry). It is an insidious disease that involves the entire body; the nervous system, digestive tract, pancreas, lungs, excretory organs, endocrine system, and the entire defense mechanisms. The frequent reoccurrence of a malignancy after treatment with the conventional methods of surgery, radiation and/or chemotherapy, results because the basic underlying metabolic cause of the cancer is rarely considered and consequently remains uncorrected[35]."

Dr Manner's final statement is most noteworthy and should be repeated and put into context. If the underlying reason cancer manifests itself is a vitamin/mineral deficiency exacerbated by a weak immune system or carcinogenic stimuli such as smoking, then of course cancer may re-occur, even after successful surgery, chemo- or radiotherapy. The reason this is thought to happen is because the underlying nutritional problem has not been corrected. Most medical doctors today receive no formal training in nutrition, educated as they are in institutions funded by pharmaceutical conglomerates promoting their own drug cures[36]. This adequately explains why many metabolic diseases are being disastrously tackled not with the required nutritional elements, but often with potent, toxic drug 'remedies'.

Philip Binzel MD, a doctor who retrained to treat his cancer patients with nutritional therapy, forgoing the dangers of toxic chemotherapy and radiation treatments, states:

---

[35] **Manner, Dr Harold W** *Metabolic Therapy in Cancer,* Cytopharma de Mexico, S.A, PO Box 434931, San Ysidro, CA 92143 USA Tel: +(52)66804371
[36] **Binzel MD, Philip** *Alive and Well,* American Media, 2000

"Most of my first patients were those who had all of the surgery, radiation and chemotherapy they could tolerate and their tumors were still growing. I did for these patients the best I knew to do.

My biggest problem at the time was understanding nutrition. In four years of medical school, one year of Family Practice residency, I had not had even one lecture on nutrition[37]."

Another side of the cancer picture that will be explained is why some people live into their eighties smoking twenty a day with no apparent ill effects. Has their diet and resultant robust immune system spared them up to now? We'll find out more as we proceed.

As already discussed, cancer researchers such as Professor John Beard of Edinburgh University and Drs. Ernst Krebs Jr. and Sr. discovered the role embryonic stem cells play in the formation of trophoblastic cells which are employed by the body in pregnancy. But it is in their additional role as 'healers' that the importance and potential cancer hazards of stem cells become known. These fibroblasts or neoblasts, as they are known, are primarily employed to repair trauma sites. These cells can transform themselves into any body-part: bone material, blood, tissue or hair depending on the particular morphogenetic stimulus they receive. When our bodies are damaged in any way, estrogen stimulates the production of these cells for healing the troubled area in the same way they form trophoblast for pregnancy. Usually pancreatic enzymes terminate this healing process upon completion of the mission. In the event that they do not, cancer tumours are the result of the ongoing 'rogue' healing process. Notice that the location of resultant cancer or trophoblastic mass is specific to the original area of damage. This too becomes important as we proceed.

For many years, cancer tumours were viewed by specialists as being 'foreign' to the body. In fact, the opposite can be said to be

---

[37] Binzel MD, Philip, ibid.

true, according to Beard and Krebs. They were curious as to why cancer existed at all if the immune system were there to repel any foreign invasion. They concluded that the immune system must not be viewing cancer as a foreign threat if the cancer commenced its existence as a healing process natural and familiar to the body.

So here we have two parts to the cancer picture: our food is minerally deficient, no matter how enticing it looks, and cancer appears to be the result of normal cellular processes that are disturbed due to depleted levels of pancreatic enzymes within our bodies. So how do external cancer-causing agents fit into this picture?

We hear much today on the subject of environmental pollutants and whether they cause cancer - we will examine some of these in two later chapters. Millions are poured into research to determine whether mobile phones, agricultural chemicals, overhead power cables, drugs, foods, paints, pesticides, asbestos, fuels, microwave ovens and hundreds of other agents are responsible for starting cancers. In spite of the Medical/Industrial Complex's strident denials in debates concerning many of these products, there can be no doubt that western societies are suffering a significantly higher percentage of cancer incidence than their Third World counterparts. Interestingly, research shows that incidences of cancer always rise along with the Gross National Product (GNP) or 'industrialisation' of nations as they develop.

Logic would compel the serious and unbiased researcher firstly to examine where cancer DOESN'T occur and then search for reasons why it is not occurring. Curiously, traditional medical research does not see the need to address this issue! Consider the following table:

Country	per capita GNP	cancer per mill[38]
Mauritius	$140	216
Sri Lanka	$225	316
Portugal	$479	1,115
USA	$3,960	1,698

Proponents of the trophoblastic thesis of cancer state that smoking, carcinogenic additives and other cancer stimuli damage our bodies and determine the site at which the healing action and resulting cancer may locate. In addition to the pancreatic enzyme/lymphocyte defence our bodies are born with, nature also uses the B17 cyanide action from our food as a secondary safeguard against cancer. However, according to the researchers we report, if our immune system is weakened through malnutrition, excessive drug toxicity or other environmental factors and B17 is not plentiful in our diet, the toxins will damage our bodies, initiating a healing reaction. Cancer may afflict us in its characteristic chronic and unchecked condition if that healing action is not halted.

Let's consider some examples to see this idea in action. If smoking were the sole cause of lung cancer, then every smoker would get lung cancer. Clearly this is not the case, although smoking is extremely harmful to health. Why are some smokers surviving and others aren't? You have to be able to explain why this is happening.

Let's examine smoking through the eyes of Beard's trophoblastic thesis: Which parts of the body are damaged through smoking? Primarily the throat and lungs. These two regions then are the sites where we would expect the body to accumulate stem cells to commence healing the damage caused by smoking. In a healthy body fed with a diet rich in organic nutrition and Vitamin B17 and low in animal protein intakes (to protect pancreatic

---

[38] World Health Organisation statistics for variances in cancer rates per capita Gross National Product for 1967-1968. An in-depth study of the phenomenon of cancer as a disease of industrialisation is covered by Robert Waller in his article: *Diseases of Civilization*, featured in *The Ecologist*, Vol. 1, No. 2, August 1970

enzymes), this healing process is routinely terminated upon completion by adequate amounts of pancreatic enzymes and the smoker may never suffer the onset of cancer. In other words, what cancerous growths the enzymes don't terminate, the B17 in the subject's food will. In a body with an inadequate immune response and doubtful nutritional backup however, the healing process may not be satisfactorily terminated. Cancer could then be the result.

Recently, research has shown that mobile phone usage may warm and damage delicate areas of the ear and brain through microwave emissions. Where then would we expect the body to attempt healing this complaint? In those regions. How would cancer manifest itself in the event that this healing process was not terminated? Site-specific tumours in the inner ear and brain.

Food carcinogens and toxic gunk deposited in our gastro-intestinal tracts through poor eating habits would be expected to damage human stomachs and colons. Radiation emissions from appliances would be expected to damage our bodies either site-specifically or in general throughout our organisms (leukemias and lymphomas). Harmful solar radiation would damage our skin, and so on. If Beard, Krebs and others are correct in their research that cancer is a rogue healing process that has not terminated upon completion of its task, then much of what we have already learned about cancer can now be properly understood.

For instance, why do more poor people in western societies die from cancer than rich people in cases where both groups have undergone similar or identical orthodox treatment? Could it be that poorer people *generally* have a poorer diet (heavy meats, cheeseburgers, pizzas, etc.), lower intakes of B17 in fruits and vegetables, and are subject to greater environmental toxicity than their richer counterparts? Why is cancer almost never found at the site where the pancreas vents its enzymes into the duodenum? Why don't tribes such as the Eskimos, Hunzas and Abkhasians, who live in isolated, non-industrialised regions and eat organically grown, pesticide-free foods, ever get cancer? These are all questions we shall be examining as we put the cancer picture together.

Ernst Krebs and others surmise that most of us in the general western populations have chronic pre-clinical cancer due to the current deficiencies in our diet. Mostly though this condition does not become clinical because it is constantly arrested by the action of our pancreatic enzymes and any cellular corruption cleared up by our immune system. However, in the cases where our organism becomes weakened by, for instance, advancing age, stress, recreational/pharmaceutical drug toxicity or inadequate nutrition, a clinical condition of cancer within us may eventually become known if the final B17 defence in our diets is absent.

Vitamin B17 is very concentrated in foods that generally no longer appear in the staple western diet, and we need to correct this immediately. Millet bread, apple and apricot seeds, the seeds of cherries, greengages, peaches and plums were all consumed by our ancestors but are rarely eaten by us today. Our great grandmothers often used to crush up the seeds and mix their piquant taste into jam preserves and sauces. Sadly this practice too has passed. Who eats the seeds of an apple or takes a nutcracker and splits open an apricot pit? What percentage of the population even eats apricots or an adequate intake of raw fruits and vegetables daily without corrupting them with heat, radiation from microwaves and pesticides from our agro-chemical industry? Is it any wonder that western populations suffer an acute shortage of the essential B17 nitrilosides and we have been reaping the whirlwind? Diets have changed over the years. Today we have the junk diet, which in reality is no fitting diet at all, and some quite real and debilitating diseases are putting in an appearance as our bodies fight and lose the battle to acquire the basic vitamins and minerals they need to maintain health.

We can learn some great basic nutrition from our animals. When our hounds become sick, do they dutifully grab our cheque books in their mouths and trot off down to the vet? No! They're out in the back yard chowing down on grasses which are plentiful in hydrocyanic acid. If you give an African Grey parrot an apple to eat, watch what he does with it. He will shred the pulp and get to the seeds first, before mopping up the mess on the floor of his cage and your carpet as soon as you let him loose into the living room!

"An apple a day keeps the doctor away," was a ringing truth in the past. This phrase has survived for centuries. Have you ever wondered why?

And They Cried "Quackery!"

Ever since Krebs' astonishing B17 breakthrough, a thick blanket of suppression and persecution has smothered laetrile and nutritional therapy. Although the main focus always seems to settle on Vitamin B17, we are going to learn that laetrile is one of several components that make up a highly effective preventative for cancer, as well as a non-toxic, dynamic treatment for all forms of the disease itself.

But incur the wrath of the establishment Vitamin B17 has successfully done. The main attacks on nutritional therapy for cancer in the United States have come through organisations closely affiliated with the pharmaceutical and chemical combines who have much to lose if a penniless vitamin and clean living ever became known by the public as the answer to cancer[39]. The attackers' list includes the Food & Drug Administration (FDA), American Cancer Society, the National Cancer Institute and investigative organisations, the American Council on Science and Health, the Consumer Health Information Research Institute, the National Council Against Health Fraud and Quackwatch Inc. These 'watchdogs' all have one goal: to cry 'quackery!' and shut down or vilify all alternative cancer treatments that threaten the gravy-train of the $11 billion cancer-drug industry[40]. Sadly, they have succeeded in America when statements like this become part of the official record:

"Because their practices fall outside of standard medical practice [in other words, because they don't burn or poison the patient with chemo- or radiotherapy], *physicians who offer unconventional cancer treatments are vulnerable to the civil charge*

---

[39] Mullins, Eustace *Murder by Injection*, ibid.

[40] **Moss, Dr Ralph W** *Questioning Chemotherapy: A Critique of the Use of Toxic Drugs in the Treatment of Cancer*, Equinox Press, 1995 ISBN 188102525X From this source, the estimated worldwide sales of all anti-cancer agents for 1997 were $11 billion. Cytotoxics (including chemos like Taxol) represented approximately $7 billion.

of malpractice." (Office of Technology United States Congress, Archive of 1990.)

I have spent considerable time investigating the claims of those who attack B17. The first noteworthy point is that the detractors cannot agree on how to 'detract'. Some attack the reputations of nutritional therapy proponents, such as Krebs, Griffin, Moss, Manner, Burk and Richardson. Some of these were deemed professional enough to attain key posts in leading medical institutions, but then apparently became complete idiots, 'quacks' and 'untrustworthy individuals' as soon as they put their careers on the line to stand behind the effectiveness of laetrile and its co-factors. One is of course tempted to ask what would possess any institution doctor to risk his enviable livelihood, reputation and income backing something that 'didn't work', an action which would probably cost him his job. What makes a man or woman do that? Something monumental maybe? Something like the truth?

Dr Benjamin Wilson wrote an article for Quackwatch Inc. implying that Ernst Krebs Jr. was an itinerant quack with fabricated qualifications: *"Ernst T. Krebs, Jr. -- Laetrile's "father" -- has often been referred to as "Dr Krebs" although he has no accredited doctoral degree. He attended Hahnemann Medical College in Philadelphia from 1938 to 1941, but was expelled after repeating his freshman year and failing his sophomore year...* [41]*"*

Our researchers were intrigued about this colourful new version of Ernst Krebs' background, so we wrote to Dr Wilson asking him to source his information. We received a reply, not from Wilson, but from Quackwatch Inc.'s chairman, Dr Stephen Barrett, who referred us to a Dr Victor Herbert. Interestingly, during the three days we waited for Dr Herbert to provide us with his sources, Dr Wilson popped up with a reply:

"I got that information from "Vitamins & 'Health' Foods: The Great American Hustle" by Herbert and Barrett, 1981; Fourth

---

[41] http://www.quackwatch.com

39

printing, 1984. George F. Stickley Company, Philadelphia. It's in Chapter 9, page 110. - B. Wilson"

Curiously we see that Stephen Barrett himself was Wilson's source, having co-wrote the book with Herbert! Our Stephen Ransom wrote back to Barrett:

"As the book was co-written by yourself, Stephen, perhaps you would be able to give me the answer? Yours, Steve Ransom."

Barrett replied: *"Sorry, I don't recall the original source. It might have been a New York Times article about laetrile written in the mid or late 1970s. You can be sure, however, that I saw appropriate documentation at the time the book was written."*

So here we have three different influential writers, affiliated to Quackwatch Inc., dipping into unsourced information, all 'apparently' correct.

Other detractors go the route that 'laetrile is cyanide'. To most who read the publications and web sites of these watchdogs, it would seem that cancerous people have indeed gone mad, ditching 'toxic chemotherapy' in favour of eating 'cyanide'. Hardly ever is the reader made aware that taking B17 in its natural form is nothing more controversial than cracking open apricot pits and eating the bitter soft seeds within. Yet, through persistent and at times downright paranoid propaganda, the little yellow apricot has become a natural-born killer in the eyes of many. Interesting also, isn't it, that the establishment is dismal in its consistency. It focuses on "Cyanide – what are you crazy?!" but fails to pillory Vitamin B12 as a 'deadly agent', as it too contains the cyanide radical (Vitamin B12 is known as <u>cyano</u>cobalomin).

Today governments protect us from 'killer B17' by outlawing the manufacturing of laetrile derived from apricot seeds, all the while sanctioning hundreds of thousands to be poisoned with chemotherapy treatments so their hair falls out, their liver and kidneys become damaged, their faces turn yellow and the cash-flow remains uninterrupted. The establishment has stopped short of depriving us completely of our apples, peaches and apricots, you'll be pleased to hear. But today, if you pass out processed laetrile in the United States of America, the Food & Drug Administration are serious about putting you in jail for trading 'a pharmaceutical' unlicensed by the FDA.

The Internet has largely been responsible for the dissemination of the laetrile story in recent years. If one searches on the word 'laetrile' on Webcrawler, one will pull up around three dozen sites. At the last go, there was only one stentorian, dissenting voice among them. Let's listen to William Jarvis MD, another Quackwatch writer, who states: *"Quackery can harm our democratic society when large numbers of people hold wrong beliefs about the nature of cancer and the best way to deal with it[42]."*

First of all, isn't it special that Jarvis recognises that large numbers of people disagree with him about the nature of cancer and the best way to deal with it! Why would they disagree if medicine were succeeding with cancer? Dr Jarvis implicitly advocates the traditional route for cancer treatment since his organisation attempts to expose any and all treatments unsanctioned by orthodox medicine. Jarvis further implies in his article, *How Quackery Harms,* that he and orthodox medicine in general have the correct belief about the nature of cancer and the best way to deal with it. Is this borne out with the ghastly cancer death rate today and the glaring inability of Jarvis' medicine to stop it? Many people, including members of my own family, have perished, not from the cancers with which they were originally diagnosed, but as a result of the toxic quackery practised on them in the name of 'cutting-edge' medicine. How many other families have lost loved ones to yellow faces and the inevitable shutting down of their livers through the extreme toxicity of prescribed cancer medications?

Ernst Krebs, Professor John Beard, Roffo, Gurchot and others were doing in-depth studies in trophoblast cells, natural nitrilosides

---

[42] **Jarvis, Dr William T** *How Quackery Harms,* http://www.quackwatch.com

and formulating their unitarian theses on B17 decades ago, and yet official medicine still maintains the naive, ignorant view that apricot seeds 'poison people', but can produce not a single genuine victim in support of its allegations. More to the point, if apricot seeds are supposed to be so lethal, why is this 'vicious' fruit still being sold in our supermarkets?

Joe Vialls: *"The American FDA bombarded the media with a story about an unfortunate couple who had poisoned themselves by eating raw apricot seeds in San Francisco. The story made headline news across the USA, although several suspicious journalists never managed to establish the identity of the unfortunate couple, despite many determined attempts[43]."*

On his web site, Jarvis lumps laetrile in with dubious alternative and New Age remedies in the hope of discrediting B17 through mockery. *"The highwayman demands 'your money OR your life'",* he trumpets. *"But quacks* [including B17 proponents] *demand your money AND your life!"* Is this not the pot calling the kettle black? What do today's orthodox cancer treatments demand, if not *'your money AND your life'*? How much are a couple of pounds of apricots anyway?

Unfortunately Jarvis also believes that when a patient is diagnosed as 'terminal', they should just accept it, go home and... well, die. Jarvis remonstrates, *"Those who accept their fate are in the best position to use their remaining time wisely."*

What a sad statement. It's a good job Dr Dale Danner from Santa Paula, California, didn't read that and go home to die. Nor William Sykes, Joe Botelho, Donald Factor, Jason Vale, Alicia Buttons and others you will meet later. The bottom line is, despite all the arguments, all the bitter invective, court cases, law suits and the slamming of jail cell doors on renegade doctors and 'vitamin

---

[43] Several attempts have been made to present 'victims' of apricot-seed poisoning to the public in an attempt to discredit B17. Like the cases above, these have been exposed as frauds. Doctors, oncologists and biochemists who support B17 therapy vigorously endorse the vitamin's harmlessness when used in accordance with researched guidelines.

smugglers', people are STILL taking B17 Metabolic Therapy for cancer and many are making startling recoveries.

My question to Dr Jarvis is simply this: "If you got cancer, what treatment would you take?" If you reply, "Chemo, x-rays or surgery", then you are definitely in the minority among your peers and probably making the statement just for the cameras. As previously stated, a survey conducted at McGill University in Montreal demonstrated that of 118 cancer doctors polled, 64 of the 79 respondents would not consent to be in a trial containing cisplatin, a common chemotherapy drug. <u>Fifty-eight found all the trials unacceptable</u>. Their reason? <u>The ineffectiveness of chemotherapy and its unacceptable degree of toxicity</u>.

By the way, who is this strident, dissenting voice and B17's *bête noire* on the Internet? Dr William Jarvis is also president of the previously mentioned National Council Against Health Fraud. Isn't that something?

The Politics of Genocide

Many are naturally uncomfortable with the idea that our governments and corporate health authorities, those supposedly watching out for us, could be embroiled in withholding the answer to cancer for commercial gain. After all, to admit to something like this would be to entertain a notion so ghastly about the kind of society in which we live, that our first reaction must be to reject such outlandish suggestions out of hand. We are often predisposed to believing the best of one another. Man is after all essentially a creature of optimism. In the case of cancer and other 'diseases' however, we'd better become realistic and pull our heads out of the sand, as the growing death statistics urge us. In this chapter, we shall examine some of the problems nutritional therapy for cancer and its pioneers have had in presenting themselves to the world stage for the benefit of all humanity.

Firstly, by way of a simple example, let us go back to the scenario surrounding smoking. For years in England, the ordinary citizen knew that if one smoked cigarettes, one would probably contract a serious disease. In other words, it was generally understood and common gossip on the street that cigarettes were harmful to a smoker's health. We did not need to be scientists to figure this out. We saw that the majority of those who smoked, coughed and most of those eventually died of that cough.

Yet we also watched bemused as expert after expert prevaricated on the subject. Two health spokesmen in America, Dr Ian MacDonald and Dr Henry Garland, defended cigarette smoking as a harmless pastime unrelated to cancer in the 1950s. MacDonald, a prominent cancer surgeon listed in *Who's Who,* even coined the phrase, *"A pack a day keeps lung cancer away[44]."*

But scientific reality about cigarettes was to tell a different story and these men were of course tragically wrong in their beliefs.

---

[44] *US News & World Report,* "Here's Another View: Tobacco May Be Harmless," 2nd August 1957, pp. 85-86

MacDonald and Garland were also the individuals who almost single-handedly buried the truth about B17 in the infamous 1953 California Report, a fraudulent document still cited today to counter the true findings on laetrile. Neither MacDonald, a prominent cancer surgeon quoted in America's *Who's Who*, nor Garland, a radiologist, had any personal experience using B17/laetrile to treat cancer patients. They had never observed its efficacy face-to-face and had a vested interest in ensuring that laetrile was discredited. Their report was highly opinionated, tarnished with scientific incompetence and later also proved to be a tragic mistake for millions. The pitiable footnote is that both doctors were later charged with accepting money under the table from the tobacco industry and ironically were ultimately to perish from their error. MacDonald was burned to death in his bed a few years later when it was believed the cigarette he had been smoking set his bedclothes on fire. Garland, who bragged that he had chain-smoked from childhood and that cigarettes were just an innocent pastime, died of lung cancer.

We also watched as the British Government dragged its heels for decades as test after test appeared to produce nothing conclusive in relation to how smoking affected a person's health, or even if it did. In the meantime millions perished of later recognised smoking-related illnesses. There was another consideration however which no doubt factored into the establishment's attitude. In the UK alone, tobacco produces billions of pounds of annual tax revenue for Her Majesty's Government.

Cancer has always been big business, but in considering how this industry is wide open to serious abuse and corruption, Dr Ralph Moss, former Assistant Director of Public Affairs at Sloan Kettering, perhaps America's foremost cancer research establishment, revealed some rather telling information on a Laurie Lee Radio Show interview in 1994:

Moss: *"About 630,000 people die every year of cancer in the US, and it really is an epidemic disease. We have got a tremendous industry. Every one of those people who is getting cancer and dying of it is going to be treated, and these treatments* *are extremely expensive. Chemo is tens of thousands, sometimes hundreds of thousands of dollars. A bone marrow transplant, which is basically another way of giving chemotherapy, or radiation, can run to about $150,000 per person, and is almost never effective. It kills about 25% of the patients."*

Lee: Why carry on doing it?

Moss: *Because of the money, which is tremendous. If you look at the board of directors at Memorial Sloan Kettering [MSK], you will find that the drug industry has a dominant position on that board. One company in particular, Bristol Myers, which produces between 40-50% of all the chemotherapy in the world, has top positions at MSK hospital.*

Lee: Doesn't that constitute a serious conflict of interest?

Moss: *They are selling their own drugs to that particular hospital but they have written into the by-laws of the center that it does not constitute a conflict of interest to sell their company drugs to the center. They get around it by not taking a salary. They are not paid, they are volunteers. Look what happens. You have men like Benno Schmidt, who was first head of the president's cancer panel under Nixon, who then becomes head at Memorial Sloan Kettering. He then goes on using the knowledge he gained at MSK to set up his own drug company to make tens of millions of dollars.*

Lee: Another revolving door?

Moss: *You bet. A big one... The American Cancer Society takes in $400 million a year. What are they doing with it? Where are the treatments? Where are the cures? Where is the good research? However the bigger thing is the industrial interest. If you look at the board of Memorial Sloan Kettering, you will find the 'Who's Who' of the petro-chemical industry. Why are they there? The emphasis is not on prevention, always on CURE. The people who are directing cancer research have a vested interest in keeping the scientists away from that area [prevention] and focused on DRUG cures, things that can be patented, marketed* *and so forth, and the US Food & Drug Administration is in total collusion in this. They have set up a system where it costs hundreds of millions of dollars to develop a new drug in America. Well, right there you know you are dealing with a monopoly situation.*

Lee: You can't be a small company and afford those research bills.

Moss: *You can't get in. It's a poker game where the ante is $100 million.... Do you know what the president of MSK makes?*

Lee: $400,000 a year?

Moss: *That's chicken feed. The president of MSK makes $2 million a year... $2.2 million.*

Evidence of special interests within the commercial cancer orbit is not hard to unearth. For instance, one of the directors of US cancer research centre Sloan Kettering is John Reed. John Reed's other job is Director of Philip Morris Tobacco Company.

As previously mentioned, pharmaceutical conglomerate Bristol-Meyers Squibb is responsible for nearly half the chemotherapy sales in the world. James Robinson was Director of BMS. His other job was Chairman of the Board of Sloan Kettering[45].

John Diamond MD and Lee Cowden MD tell us that *"Cancer research has been set up almost entirely in favor of conventional approaches ever since the war on cancer, formalized in 1971 as the National Cancer Act, was first scripted in the 1960s. At that time, Senator Ralph Yarborough (D-Texas) organized the National Panel of Consultants of the Conquest of Cancer. Of its 26 members, 10 came from the American Cancer Society and 4 were affiliated with Memorial Sloan Kettering Hospital. Benno Schmidt, MD, the director of Sloan Kettering's Cancer Center, was the*

---

[45] *Gulliver's* magazine, fall 1997 (212) 730-5433

panel's chairman. Sidney Farber, MD, former president of the ACS [American Cancer Society], was its vice chairman[46]."

Today, cancer-related expenditures are about $1/9^{th}$ of the overall health budget in the United States and, according to American Cancer Society figures, total cancer expenditures, directly and indirectly, for hospitals, doctors, nurses, oncologists, research, etc. total over $100 billion a year. It isn't hard to see a strong economic dynamic determining how this budget is allocated, and to whom.

When news of Vitamin B17's startling effect in treating cancers through nutritional therapy spread throughout America, the pharmaceutical companies and orthodox medical establishment were compelled to answer the claims made by the laetrilists. Attempts were made, through deceitful wording, to refer to Vitamin B17 as 'a drug', which naturally meant laetrile had to be licensed before its official use could be sanctioned. Of course, powerful interests within the government, research facilities and pharmaceutical combines had not the slightest intention of sanctioning a penniless vitamin that could not be patented and sold for huge profit in the fight against cancer. Dr John Heinerman explains what happened next:

"When President Richard Nixon was deluged with tens of thousands of petitions from ordinary citizens everywhere demanding clinical trials for laetrile, these demands were forwarded to his cancer advisor, Benno Schmidt... When Schmidt consulted all of his medical colleagues about laetrile, he found them vehemently opposed to it. But, interestingly enough, as he told reporters later: "I couldn't get anybody to show me scientific proof that the stuff didn't work[47].""

Nevertheless, wishing to be seen by the public to test laetrile 'on a level playing field', the establishment commissioned several

[46] Diamond, Dr John and Dr Lee Cowden, ibid.
[47] **Heinerman, Dr John** *An Encyclopedia of Nature's Vitamins and Minerals*, Prentice Hall, 1998 ISBN 0735200726

studies, including a 1953 project at Stanford University, a 1961 study at UC Berkeley, one in 1962 at the Diablo Laboratories in Berkeley and a 1965 trial on behalf of the Canadian Medical Association at McGill University in Montreal.

In 1973 a three-month trial at the Southern Research Institute in Birmingham, Alabama, intensively researched the therapeutic properties of laetrile. The institute finally released its findings to the National Cancer Institute which proceeded to announce to the public that once again studies proved that B17 had no effect whatsoever in the treatment of cancer. However not all was as it appeared. When the data and protocols from these experiments were subsequently studied in more detail by an honest Dr Dean Burk, one of the National Cancer Institute's founders and head of its Department of Cytochemistry, inconsistencies began to appear[48].

Author Edward Griffin explains: *"Every study had been tarnished with the same kind of scientific ineptitude, bias, and outright deception as found in the 1953 MacDonald/Garland California report. Some of these studies openly admitted evidence of anti-cancer effect but hastened to attribute this effect to other causes. Some were toxicity studies only, which means that they weren't trying to see if laetrile was effective, but merely to determine how much of it was required to kill the patient[49]."*

Despite announcing to the world that laetrile was useless, the National Cancer Institute, the American Medical Association and the drug companies looked on with anger as a national grass-roots movement sprang up across America as a result of the many cancer recoveries being reported and attributed to nutritional therapy. It was the '70s and people were distrustful of their

---

[48] Dean Burk, Ph.D, one of the National Cancer Institute's co-founders, endorsed B17's status as a true vitamin and offered this statement regarding Edward Griffin's *World Without Cancer*: *"A clear and revolutionary insight into both the science and politics of cancer therapy."* Dr Linus Pauling, the 'father' of Vitamin C and two-time Nobel Laureate (the only man in Nobel history to win the same prize twice), also supported the use of laetrile (*The New England Journal of Medicine*, 8th July 1982)

[49] Griffin, G Edward, ibid.

government as a result of Watergate and Vietnam. The Committee for Freedom-of-Choice in Cancer Therapy was formed, founding several hundred chapters across America which in turn held public meetings, press conferences and pressured state legislative committees into calling for the 'legalisation' of Vitamin B17.

By way of an answer, the National Cancer Institute launched yet another trial to debunk laetrile in 1978. This time, the records of laetrile-treated cancer patients were mixed in with those treated with conventional therapy and the panel not notified which cases received which treatment. Judgement was to be based on therapy 'results'. In determining which yardstick to use in order to gauge the effectiveness of the patient's treatment, it was finally decided to use tumour shrinkage. The problem with judging the success of a trial using this method is that most tumours only contain a small percentage of cancer cells. And while chemotherapy may reduce tumours by as much as 60% in some cases but not rid the patient of the cancer, laetrile will target only the malignant cancer cells, but reduce the tumour much less. As Griffin remarks: *"[In most B17 trials] a living and healthy patient with a tumour reduced by only 15% would be classified a failure. A sick and dying patient with a tumour reduced 60% would be a success."*[50]

To traditional oncology the tumour is the cancer. Thus when a tumour is removed or burned away, the patient receives an 'all-clear', with of course the traditional reservations. The problem is, according to Krebs and Beard, the tumour is not the cause of the cancer, merely the symptom of it. If the tumour is removed, what about the proposed root cause of the cancer – nutritional deficiency and environmental/food toxins? Did the doctors dislodge trophoblast cells which later migrated to metastasise (spread) at other locations, once the estrogen got to them? How will these cells be killed if the root cause of the cancer is not addressed? Very commonly, as we know, secondary cancers flare up and are almost impossible to defeat. When radiation is applied to some tumours, they can under certain circumstances actually accelerate! This makes perfect sense, if you consider that the radiation is

---

[50] Griffin, G Edward, ibid.

hurting the patient, whose body then proceeds to produce more healing trophoblast.

The panel found the following results from the 22 laetrile cases it examined:

2 patients demonstrated complete response (tumours disappeared)
4 patients experienced partial tumour regression in excess of 50%
9 patients experienced stability of tumour size (no further growth)
3 patients had "increased disease-free intervals"

And so 18 out of 22 cancer cases, when judged on tumour size, showed a marked response to laetrile even though tumour reduction is largely incidental to laetrile's *modus operandi*. This 82% response rate cannot be matched, even closely, by ANY conventional cancer therapy today, yet this is not even the fairest method of recording the effectiveness of nutritional therapy!

But once again, B17 was to be grotesquely misrepresented. The Establishment's panel made its determination and laetrile was 'tossed under the bus' with the report's incredible conclusion: *"These results allow no definite conclusion supporting the anti-cancer activity of laetrile."*

Meanwhile cancer specialist Dr Harold Manner had not been idle. While the controversy raged around him, he and his team of graduate students at Loyola University, Chicago were studying the effects of laetrile/amygdalin when combined with the enzymes pancreatin, trypsin, papain and bromelain combined with Vitamins A and E in their emulsified form. Manner contended that laetrile and the vitamins would not produce noticeable anti-cancer results without the cancer 'shell' coating first being weakened or destroyed by these enzymes. The natural action of pancreatic enzymes within our bodies is to weaken and digest the protein coating of trophoblast cells, allowing the body's immune system lymphocytes to destroy the cells.

Manner's results were published and broadcast in a series of press conferences. His exotic findings were met with a wall of indignation and denial from his peers. At the same time the

Chicago doctor was broadcasting his startling results on his combined vitamin/enzyme/laetrile protocol, a major study on laetrile was being undertaken at the Rockefeller institute of Sloan Kettering Memorial Hospital in New York. Many laetrile cynics believed that the object of these trials was once again to demonstrate to the public that B17 was useless in treating cancer and that conventional therapy was the only game in town.

Dr Kanematsu Sugiura was chosen as the director of this five-year study. With over 60 years' experience in research, rising in the ranks to senior researcher of one of the world's most prestigious cancer research institutions, Dr Sugiura's work was trusted and his honesty and integrity admired and unquestioned by all. This naturally made him a disastrous choice as head of a study in which the object of the exercise was apparently to suppress the truth about B17's cancer-treating abilities. No one has been able adequately to explain why Dr Sugiura was chosen for this trial at all. His final report was to prove a monumental embarrassment to Memorial Sloan Kettering and the monied corporate powers which funded it.

The conclusions of Sugiura's five-year examination were these:

1. Laetrile inhibited the growth of tumours
2. It stopped the spreading (metastasising) of cancer in mice
3. It relieved pain
4. It acted as a cancer preventative
5. It improved general health

His official report read as follows: *"The results clearly show that amygdalin significantly inhibits the appearance of lung metastases in mice bearing spontaneous mammary tumors and increases significantly the inhibition of the growth of primary tumors...*

Laetrile also seems to prevent slightly the appearance of new tumors... The improvement of health and appearance of the treated animals in comparison to the controls is always a common observation. Dr Sugiura has never observed complete regression of these tumors on all his cosmic experience with other chemotherapeutic agents."

Ironically it took a while for the implications of Sugiura's findings to sink into the Sloan Kettering boardroom. Two colleagues of Sugiura's had also duplicated his findings with amygdalin. Dr Elizabeth Stockert and Dr Lloyd Schoen, both biochemists based at MSK, verified Sugiura's consistent findings, Schoen even obtaining a 100% cure rate among Swiss albino mice with Manner's additional proteolytic enzyme supplements - later to become a common co-procedure among laetrile physicians and the basis for the B17 Metabolic Therapy we recognise today.

Up to this point, Sugiura's work had never been questioned. In fact in 1962, hundreds of the well-respected Japanese researcher's papers were published in a four-volume set, the following introduction to the collective works glowingly penned by Dr C Chester Stock, head of Sloan Kettering's testing division:

"Few if any names in cancer research are as widely known as Kanematsu Sugiura's... Possibly the highest regard in which his work is held is best characterized by a comment made to me by a visiting investigator in cancer research from Russia. He said, "When Dr Sugiura publishes, we know we don't have to repeat the study, for we would obtain the same results he has reported.""

But the most well respected cancer researcher in America had just vindicated B17! The truth of the situation suddenly hit Sloan Kettering and the drug companies like a sledgehammer. To make matters worse, the findings of Drs Sugiura, Schoen and Stockert were already a matter of public record and had attracted the undivided attentions of the media.

Sloan Kettering and the cancer industry reacted in the only way they knew how. Sugiura's reputation notwithstanding, more trials were immediately sanctioned. While no one outright insulted Sugiura's research abilities, statements released by MSK implied that some procedures may have been bungled. Had the directors of Sloan Kettering begun to realise that Sugiura's allegiance lay more with the truth of his findings than with Sloan Kettering's political and financial considerations? With the public spotlight fixed firmly upon them and the cancer industry's cash-flow up for debate, the latter realised they could not ask Dr Sugiura to stand down, and so were compelled to involve the Japanese researcher in a limited role in the trials that followed.

Soon after, certain employees at Sloan Kettering began to recognise Dr Sugiura's findings on laetrile were being deliberately obfuscated. Several prominent staff-members became enraged. To the great embarrassment of MSK's board of directors, an anonymously-written newsletter entitled *Second Opinion* mysteriously appeared. Its accurate information detailed Sugiura's findings, complete with photocopies of hand-written lab reports listing the Center's experimental results on laetrile, test by test, mouse by mouse. The reports plainly exposed the on-going research cover-up. Appalled Center officials recognised that the leak obviously originated from within the Manhattan medical institution. Key media contacts and laetrile advocates were top of *Second Opinion's* mailing list and received full details. The press licked its lips, sensing a major coup in the making.

In the meantime, Dr Sugiura was involved in repeated follow-up trials as Sloan Kettering provided him with successive research partners, each of whom seemed desperate to override him and prove laetrile was useless in the treatment of cancer. Sugiura by now recognised the sinister power play in operation. On 15th June 1977, a news conference was convened at Sloan Kettering to announce the conclusion of the laetrile trials. All the big guns from the institution attended, as did the press. Dr Sugiura was also called to attend but forbidden from taking part.

Dr Robert Good, President of the Center, rose to his feet and announced that *"After careful and exhaustive testing, laetrile was found to possess neither preventative, nor tumor-regressant, nor anti-metastatic, nor curative anti-cancer activity."*

"Dr Sugiura!" someone suddenly shouted. *"Do you stick by your belief that laetrile stops the spread of cancer?"*

The room suddenly became very quiet as the cameras turned on the elderly Japanese doctor for his reaction. Dr Sugiura, one of the world's most highly respected and experienced cancer researchers, calmly looked the reporter in the eye and, in a clear voice, replied, *"I stick!"*

The following month, in July 1977, government hearings were held before the Subcommittee on Health and Scientific Research under Senator Edward Kennedy. The title of the published report was, "Banning of the Drug Laetrile from Interstate Commerce by the Food & Drug Administration". Dr Lewis Thomas, President of Sloan-Kettering, testified at the hearing:

"There is not one particle of scientific evidence to suggest that laetrile possesses any anti-cancer properties at all. I am not aware of any scientific papers, published in any of the world's accredited journals of medical science, presenting data in support of the substance, although there are several papers, one of these recently made public by Sloan Kettering Institute, reporting the complete absence of anti-cancer properties in a variety of experimental animals."

In that one statement, made before the representatives of the American people in 1977, Dr Lewis Thomas buried the 'drug' laetrile and took away from his countrymen the legal right to obtain supplies to heal themselves of cancer with the proven and tested action of a simple vitamin.

G Edward Griffin: *"The directors and officers at Sloan Kettering continued to denigrate Dr Sugiura's findings, claiming that no one else had ever been able to duplicate them. In other words, they lied. Not only did they lie, they did so on a subject that directly affects the lives of hundreds of thousands of cancer victims each year. It is not an exaggeration to say that over a million people have needlessly gone to their deaths as a result of that lie. There is a word for that. It is genocide[51]."*

---

[51] Griffin, G Edward, ibid. Also **Griffin, G Edward** *Private Papers Relating to Laetrile*, American Media, 1997 ISBN 0912986204

I was interviewed on a radio show in Salt Lake City in October 2000 and was quizzed about these events at Sloan Kettering. After I had explained to the listeners what had happened at the institution, the radio show host asked a doctor, also on the program, whether this was true. The doctor in question stated that he had been working at Sloan Kettering at the time and indeed Sugiura had been deliberately censored.

Dr Ralph Moss was the Assistant Director of Public Affairs at Sloan Kettering during most of the events in question. Pressure was put on Moss to write the press release claiming that laetrile was ineffective. Ultimately on 17th November 1977, Moss went public and convened a press conference of his own at the Hilton Hotel in Manhattan, NY. Admitting that he had been one of the authors of *Second Opinion*, Dr Moss charged that Memorial Sloan Kettering was guilty of a huge scientific fraud and cover-up, producing documentation and naming names in support of his allegations. Not surprisingly he was fired from the institution the following day. In his radio interview on the Laurie Lee Show in 1994, Dr Ralph Moss discussed his position and opinions on Dr Sugiura's findings and their implications:

Moss: *Shortly after I went to work* [at the Sloan Kettering Cancer Institute], *I went to visit an elderly Japanese scientist, Kanematsu Sugiura, who astonished me when he told me he was working on laetrile (B17). At the time it was the most controversial thing in cancer, reputed to be a cure for cancer.*

We in Public Affairs were giving out statements that laetrile was worthless, it was quackery, and people should not abandon proven therapies. I was astonished that our most distinguished scientist would be bothering with something like this, and I said, "Why are you doing this if it doesn't work?" He took down lab books and showed me that in fact laetrile was dramatically effective in stopping the spread of cancer. The animals were genetically programmed to get breast cancer and about 80-90% of them normally get a spread of cancer from the breast to the lungs which is a common route in humans. When they gave the animals laetrile

56

by injection, only 10-20% of them got lung metastases. And these facts were verified by many people, including the Center's pathology department.

Lee: So this is verified, that laetrile can have this positive effect?

Moss: *We were finding this and yet we in Public Affairs were told to issue statements to the exact opposite of what we were finding scientifically. As the years went by, I got more wrapped up in this thing and three years later I said all this in my own press conference, and was fired the next day "for failing to carry out his most basic job responsibility."*

The writing of history always goes to the victor. Legislation was subsequently passed banning the interstate commerce of laetrile/amygdalin B17 for the treatment of cancer in America. Today, thousands of cancer sufferers, unwilling to undergo the punishing and expensive courses of surgery, chemo- and radiotherapy for their condition, are compelled to travel to Mexico, Germany, the UK and elsewhere in order to receive nutritional therapy treatment for their condition.

The True Face of the Corporate Agenda

Here are some of the lies that have cost you your loved ones...

Dr Schmidt, FDA Commissioner, in March 1974: *"...Every study to date has not found any evidence of efficacy* [with laetrile and] *if there was one shred of evidence from animal or cell systems I would issue an IND."* (Investigational New Drug status that approves clinical testing in humans)

"No evidence of anti-tumour activity has been found in any of the tests [with laetrile]*."* Robert Wetherell, Acting Director, Office of Legislative Services, US Food & Drug Administration

"All [laetrile] *testing by the National Cancer Institute has found no evidence of activity against cancer."* Dr Robert Hadsell, Office of Cancer Communications, National Cancer Institute in a letter sent throughout the US and abroad

"[laetrile] *has repeatedly been tested in animal tumour systems at the National Cancer Institute. In no instance did laetrile have activity in any animal tumour system. There is no basis for the use of laetrile in man based on the data derived from experiments in animals."* Interoffice memo sent to department heads of the US Mayo Clinic, Rochester, MN, January 1974

"Extensive animal tumour studies conducted independently at two outstanding cancer research centers, New York Memorial Sloan Kettering (MSK) and the Southern Research Institute, have shown this drug to be totally without evidence of anti-cancer activity." Dr Charles Moertel, Mayo Clinic, in a letter published in the *Rochester* (MN) *Post Bulletin*, 21st January 1974

* * * *

The National Cancer Institute's Dr Dean Burk oversaw many of the details surrounding the testing of laetrile in the 1970s. Burk states that positive, statistically highly significant, anti-cancer activity by laetrile in animal tumour systems has been observed in at least 5 independent institutions in 3 widely separated countries of the world, with a variety of animal cancers:

1). Southern Research Institute (Birmingham Alabama), for the NCI, in a majority of 280 BDF1 mice bearing Lewis lung cancers, treated with up to 400 mg Laetrile (Amygdalin MF) per kg body weight, with respect to increased median life span (3rd December 1973)

2). Sloan Kettering (New York) with CD8 F1 mice bearing spontaneous mammary carcinomas, inhibition of formation of lung metastases, inhibition of growth of primary tumours, and greater health and appearance of animal hosts, upon treatment with 1-2 gm Laetrile/per kg body weight/day. (13th June 1973)

3). Scind Laboratories, University of San Francisco, 400 rats bearing Walker 256 carcinoma (200 treated with Amygdalin, 200 controls), with 80% increase in life span at optimum dosage (500 mg Amygdalin/kg body weight). (10th Oct 1968)[52]

NCI Director Carl Baker wrote to Congressman Edwin W Edwards on 26th January 1971: *"The data provided by the McNaughton Foundation certainly indicates some activity in animal tumour systems."* (our emphasis added)

4). Pasteur Institute (Paris), with human cancer strain maintained in mice, treated at optimal dosage of 500 mg Amygdalin Marsan/kg body weight/day, increased life span and delayed tumour growth up to 100% (6th December 1971)

5). Institute Von Ardenne (Dresden, Germany), H strain mice bearing *Ehrlich ascites carcinoma* treated with bitter almond amygdalin *ad libitum* in addition to regular chow diet, yielded increased life span and decreased rate of cancer growth, treatment

---

[52] *cf.* FDA-IND 6734 application, pp. 247-248, 00080-00093

beginning 15 days before cancer inoculation (arch. Geschwulstorsch. 42, 135-7 (1973))

Dr Harold Manner, the Chicago cancer specialist, had himself verified the theoretical action of amygdalin with repeated experiments of his own. Here is an excerpt of an interview with MOTHER associate editor Bruce Woods, reprinted in the *Cancer Control Journal, Vol 6, Nos. 1-6*:

WOODS: *Can you give us some background on your Laetrile research? How did you proceed in the beginning?*

DR MANNER: *Well, as you know, Krebs suggested that Laetrile - when injected into the body - circulates through the system until it comes into contact with an enzyme capable of releasing the cyanide that the substance contains. As the theory goes, that particular enzyme - beta-glucosidase - is abundant in tumor tissue. Of course, the cyanide which the tumor triggers the Laetrile into releasing could then escape into healthy tissue and be dangerous to the entire body, but there is another enzyme in all normal tissue called rhodanese. And this enzyme neutralizes the cyanide... which is then excreted in the urine.*

That's the theory we wanted to evaluate. So we checked out the enzymes first... to determine whether or not they were where Krebs said they'd be. And, in general, we found that the highest levels of the cyanide-unlocking enzymes were in the tumorous tissue. At that point we had to find out if the Laetrile broke down as Krebs had predicted it would. So we injected the substance into mice and collected urine samples for 24 hours... to check for the sodium thiocyanate and hippuric acid that are the non-toxic end products of broken-down Laetrile.

WOODS: *And were these substances present in the urine?*

DR MANNER: *Yes, and we observed an increase in these compounds as we increased the Laetrile dosage. All of our results were reported in the scientific journals.*

What is one to make of such dissension in the ranks? If the laetrile/vitamin/enzyme protocol were useless and the open-and-shut case we are led to believe, these and many other conflicting arguments made by professionals with the most to lose make no sense whatsoever. Could the motive of laetrilists possibly be money? Who's ever going to become rich peddling apricot seed extract and enzymes to a grateful public?

"No iota of activity? NO SHRED OF EVIDENCE?" an outraged Dr Burk thundered to the enemies of laetrile. *"It will be interesting to see if FDA Commissioner Schmidt will indeed soon back up his word about issuing a laetrile IND.* [53]*"*

Laetrile/amygdalin never got its IND... and then the purges began.

California, 1990: Agents from the Food & Drug Administration burst into a pet store owned by Sissy Harrington-McGill. They arrest her for violating the Health Claims Law by declaring in her pet store literature that vitamins prolong life and improve health in pets. The fact that the Health Claims Law was never passed by Congress appeared incidental to the armed agents who haul Ms Harrington-McGill before a judge who summarily convicts her without honouring her constitutional request for a jury trial. Ms Harrington-McGill spends 114 days in jail before being released with a criminal record[54].

David Halpern, along with members of his family and the presidents of three European supplement and vitamin companies, is charged by the FDA with importing banned nutritional supplements into America. Such products are freely available in Britain and Europe's health food stores at this time. The

---

[53] Test data published in *Cancer News Journal* Vol 9, no 3. Source: The Arlin J. Brown Inf. Center, Inc, PO Box 251, Fort Belvoir, VA 22060. 703 451 8638. Tel: 540 752 9511. E mail: cancerinfo@webtv.net

[54] **Wright Legal Defense Fund** *FDA Versus the People of the United States*, Citizens For Health, PO Box 368, Tacoma, WA 98401, (206)922-2457

indictments carry with them collective prison terms totalling 990 years[55].

1992, Texas: Over a dozen major health food stores are raided by the Texas Department of Health and the Texas Department of Food and Drug, under guidance from the FDA. 'Contraband' substances such as Vitamin C, zinc, flaxseed oil, aloe vera and herbs are bagged up and hauled off by armed agents. The resulting public outrage only prompts aggressive FDA officials to corner health store owners, warning them, "Don't talk to the press, or we'll come down on you twice as hard." No charges are ever filed by the FDA against those arrested and, as usual, no products or assets are ever returned.

Probably the most celebrated early case involving the suppression of laetrile was that of 58-year-old Wichita, Kansas farmer, Glen L Rutherford. Diagnosed with cancer of the rectum in 1971, Rutherford elected to travel to Tijuana, Mexico for laetrile treatment after orthodox treatments proved ineffective. Rutherford was evidently healed of his cancer and returned to the United States where he continued to obtain laetrile from a source within his own country.

When agents of the Food & Drug Administration arrested this apparently 'illegal' source, Rutherford went to war. Bringing a class action suit against the FDA for interfering with his constitutional rights, he stormed into action in the US District Court in Kansas City, thundering at the medical authorities across the courtroom: *"You set yourselves up as God and Jesus Christ all in one!"* His righteous fury drew loud applause and howls of approbation from supporters in the public gallery. *"If I lost my laetrile, you would read my obituary in eight to ten months!"* he continued shouting. *"Give me the right to choose the way I want to die. It is not your prerogative to tell me how, only God can tell me that!"*

---

[55] **Wicke, Dr Roger** *Stop FDA's Attempts to Restrict Availability of Natural Products,* http://rmhiherbal.org/a/f.ahr6.fda.html

When physicians stood to give evidence against laetrile, testifying that it was "sugar-coated cyanide", they were drowned out by loud booing and hissing from the courtroom audience. The case dragged on for some years before a federal judge in Oklahoma City named Luther Bohanon finally ruled in favour of Rutherford, stating in his opinion dated 8th April 1977 that

"...many intelligent... citizens... have made a... decision... to employ an unproven and largely unrespected treatment in an effort to comfort, if not save, lives that orthodox [medicine] tells them have already been lost. They do so with an acute awareness of professional medicine's assessment of their choice. Their decision should be respected."

Respect or not, the hounding continued. Today Multi-Jurisdictional Task Force 'commandos' are getting in on vitamin busts to enforce the FDA's total ban on interstate commerce involving B17 laetrile and other remedies.

Roger Wicke Ph.D. reports: *"In 1993 dozens of natural healing clinics, health food stores and natural product manufacturers throughout the United States were assaulted by combined forces from the FDA, the Drug Enforcement Agency, the Internal Revenue Service, US Customs and the US Postal Service in commando-style SWAT raids. Stocks of vitamins and herbs were confiscated as well as bank accounts, automobiles, and computers. Especially of interest as a target for the raids were mailing lists of customers and clients. The Postal Service assisted in the actions by blocking all mail to some businesses, effectively preventing them from continuing any business or conducting effective legal defense[56]."*

In 1991, a cancer victim who had healed himself with non-orthodox treatments was kidnapped from his office in a Mexican hospital in Tijuana where he had set up a clinic to help others. Jimmy Keller's abduction occurred at the hands of bounty hunters employed by the US Justice Department. When returned to the United States, Keller was charged and convicted of wire fraud

[56] Wicke, Roger, ibid. See also **DeMeo, James** *Anti-Constitutional Activities and Abuse of Police Power*, http://id.mind.net/community/orgonelab/fda.htm.

(soliciting business by telephone to attract cancer victims to his clinic in Mexico) and sentenced to two years in prison.

In August 2000, the FDA and Justice Department swung into action again. John Taylor's 'enforcers' began raiding companies selling Vitamin B17 metabolic therapy kits to clinics, hospitals and members of the public worldwide. NorthWest Cable News carried the article on the web on 6th September 2000: *Experts Warn Against Laetrile on Net*. The article went on to pillory laetrile as a 'quack' remedy that could cause cyanide poisoning. The same day, CNN was also reporting: *US Aims to Stop Sale of Unapproved Cancer Remedy...* with much the same editorial input. Laetrile was cyanide for goodness sake! It was hazardous, according to the FDA, and completely useless in the treatment of cancer.

Interestingly, while all this was going on, scientists at Imperial College, Kensington, London, were slapping each other on the back, wondering who was in line for the Nobel Prize, as a team under Dr Mahendra Deonarain had just figured out a way to kill cancer cells selectively using... cyanide!

Cyanide Used to Kill Cancer Cells trumpets the *London Times*, 7th September, 2000 (page 10):

"British scientists have harnessed the deadly properties of cyanide to kill cancer cells, raising the prospect of a revolutionary drug... When the altered yeast [rich in Vitamin B17] *is added to cancer cells, it binds to them and kills them by generating cyanide, but does not affect healthy cells. Should any cyanide escape the tumours into the bloodstream, it would be rapidly broken down in the liver and neutralised."*

Amazing when you consider that this has been a matter of public record for over 50 years! This would be funny, were it not for the fact that the fraud surrounding the release of life-saving empirical data on laetrile has been suppressed and countless lives lost as a result.

Killing Cancer With Cyanide blares the Telegraph, Britain's leading broadsheet newspaper, on 7th September 2000, page 14. *"We can target any kind of cancer cell!"* Dr Deonarain triumphantly announces.

The BBC had the drop on the papers however, reporting the story as far back as April 1999, extolling the virtues of tapioca, the school dinner food made from the tropical plant cassava (rich in B17). At the time, the revered British media institution reported on the work of Professor Monica Hughes of Newcastle University. Her stated aim with the use of cassava... *"is for the cancer cells to produce hydrogen cyanide in high enough doses so that they commit suicide."*[67]

Death By Tapioca. Imagine that.

Several times during my 2000 'Straight Talk' tour, I was interviewed on American TV, on two occasions by NBC affiliates, on the subject of nutritional treatments for cancer. NBC, which has reported in the past on 'wicked' laetrile, demonstrated a remarkable lack of sensitivity to their inconsistent reporting when their web-site reported on 6th September: *Could Cyanide be Next Cancer-Killer?* Their subsequent article covered the Deonarain story from Imperial College, UK.

What a monumental embarrassment to the FDA. And all the while the US government agency slams 'wicked' cyanide as a quack cancer treatment, on 27th September 2000, InteliHealth announces that the FDA has just approved arsenic as a cancer therapy![58] The unmistakable message to the American public from the FDA appears to be: "Forget cyanide, it's dangerous quackery, for goodness sake. Here, take arsenic instead."

Such actions are the strongest evidence that the FDA's official task of protecting the American public from unsafe drugs and foodstuffs appears secondary to quelling any and all opposition to the interests of the pharmaceutical cartels who continue to operate

---

[57] BBC News (web), 12th April 1999
[58] InteliHealth Health News, 27th September 2000 – www.intelihealth.com

their billion-dollar businesses to huge profits, no matter the ethics of the methods involved.

G Edward Griffin: *"Therefore - and mark this well - as long as the present laws remain, the only substances that ever will be "approved" for cancer therapy will be proprietary. No substance from nature will ever be legally available for cancer or any other disease unless its source can be monopolised or its processing can be patented. No matter how safe and effective it may be, and no matter how many people are benefited, it will forever be relegated to the category of "unproven" therapies. As such, freely available cures from nature will always be illegal to prescribe, to promote, and in many cases even to use[59]."*

In 1982, Dr Richard Crout of the FDA made his agency's position extremely clear:

"I never have and never will approve a new drug to an individual, but only to a large pharmaceutical firm with unlimited finances."

---

[59] G Edward Griffin, ibid.

The Natural Way

"Most of what you have heard over your lifetime about [orthodox] cancer treatments is not the truth. At the very least, you have received an incomplete picture. If you believe the propaganda you have been fed and you develop cancer, it can cost you your life[60]." John Diamond MD

In many ways the abominable story of corporate cancer is the same as AIDS and other 'afflictions' that have become so newsworthy today[61]. In most cases, outright lies, fraud and deception are the agenda, but the public may take heart that these 'terrible scourges' to humanity are eminently defeatable and are indeed daily being defeated, despite what we read in the newspapers.

We saw the harrowing pictures of King Hussein of Jordan, overcome with cancer, coming to America to receive 'the latest in cancer therapies' for his condition. All the king's money and all the king's men were on offer, his jets singing on the tarmac on standby to fly him to any destination in the world where the hope of extending his life might reside, but what did King Hussein's enormous wealth buy him in the end? The bald head, sallow complexion and haunted demeanour of the brave old warrior gazing pitifully out of our TVs said it all. Cut, slash and burn allopathics. He died soon after.

Thankfully the human body with which God blessed us did not come with a packet of pills with an FDA approval stamp on it. Long before old JD, Morris Fishbein, the American Medical Association, Dr William Jarvis and insurance companies succeeded in convincing us we couldn't do without them, the human body had decent, nutritious food available to it and a T-cell lymphocyte system working away behind the scenes to return us to health if we got sick.

---

[60] Diamond, Dr John, ibid.
[61] Day, Phillip & Steven Ransom, *World Without AIDS*, ibid.

A few weeks ago I pulled my Nissan into a petrol station to fill up. I was somewhat preoccupied with my thoughts and proceeded to pump 40 litres of diesel into my gasoline vehicle. My mistake only became evident a mile up the road when my car began smoking Brixton to a standstill and some rather alarming knocking sounds issued from the sharp end. 24 hours and a £180 towing/repair bill later, I had solidly learned two very valuable lessons: one, that green means unleaded, and two, my vehicle runs better on the right kind of fuel.

And so do we. If we want to enjoy good health, then the right gas has to go in the machine. Step on the mines, smoke, eat junk, indulge in all those vain imaginations, and each of us can have a $35,000 joint replacement procedure, an amputation, lung or colorectal cancer and a triple heart-bypass operation - all paid for courtesy of the National Health or Blue Shield.

The good life is the natural life. Most of the ills the body faces while living on a good diet are known as self-limiting because the body takes care of them eventually.

We briefly looked at the immune system earlier. Steven Ransom comments: *"Fifty years ago, very little was known about our immune system. It was known that there were cells in the blood that helped to defend the body against disease, but what these cells did and how they did it was a mystery. Today immunology is a whole science and knowledge of the body's defence systems is growing all the time. Along with the red cells carrying oxygen, and big white cells that fight any foreign germs they can find, the blood stream carries millions of little round white cells called lymphocytes. T lymphocytes which originate in the thymus gland and B lymphocytes from the bone marrow are just two of the highly organised battalions of germ killers that make up the army defending us from infectious attack*[62].*"*

---

[62] **Ransom, Steven** *Homoeopathy: What Are We Swallowing?* Credence Publications, London, 1999 ISBN 0953501213

Dr Paul Brand has made a tremendous study of the intricate workings of the human body. In his work, *The Forever Feast,* Brand introduces us to the highly organised and uncompromising army that fights microbiological invaders within our bodies:

"I must share just one facet of the skills of the T lymphocytes, because I get excited at the ingenuity that must have gone into their design, and because I'm so happy to have these little guys on my side when I am sick. My T lymphocytes concentrate in places where most germs try to get into the body. It is never very long before an invading germ meets a T lymphocyte.

The first wonderful thing is that the lymphocyte knows at once that this living cell is not 'one of us', it is an enemy. The next wonderful thing is what it does. It inspects the enemy cell and takes a template or pattern of its surface, noting especially the weak points. Then our friend runs back to the factory where new cells are made and announces the emergency: "An enemy has entered the body and is rapidly multiplying. We have to manufacture antibodies of exactly this shape, so that the enemy will be killed and no other cell will be harmed."

An older lymphocyte may hurry up at this point and tell the factory that the shape of the needed antibodies is exactly the size as was used a year ago, when there was a brief war in the body during the flu season. Therefore there is no need to repeat the time-consuming preparation of the prototype antibodies - we already have them. All that is needed is to rush into mass production. Thus before the virus has time to do any real harm, masses of specific antibodies are all over the body, overcoming every last virus and restoring health and wholeness everywhere[63]."

This means that in more cases than we care to admit, our bodies will heal themselves in due course, given rest, proper nutrition, de-stressed surroundings and *no therapeutic intervention*. Yes, of course there are exceptions and a doctor should always be consulted when in doubt. But mankind must learn to exercise a

---

[63] **Brand, Dr Paul** *The Forever Feast*, Monarch Publications, 1994

little discretion when it comes to swallowing everything Nurse shoves down its throat. There is a happy, mature and sensible middle ground, and one which will save us money, unimaginable grief and lead to a much happier and more stress-free life.

Once again we must remind ourselves of accredited research, such as Ralph Nader's 300,000 Americans killed every year through negligent medical and prescription procedures - and that's before the nutritional diseases get us. Have cancer, AIDS, Alzheimer's, ME (chronic fatigue), MS, and Parkinson's really been killing us, or have we not signed our own death warrants yet again with a lackadaisical disregard for the truth about what our bodies really need and what drugs and environmental factors will eventually do us in[64]?

Cancer is a parable that tells how mankind's wonderful technology gave us cheap new convenience foods, stripped of goodness, and great new chemical products, packed with carcinogens, which began to kill us. I have watched 'AIDS' and cancer patients in my own family die through historically deadly drug and radiation therapy even after being told what made them sick and what could make them better. Incredibly they never even bothered to read the information they were given. Why? Because even when faced with their own impending death, they could not bring themselves to end their worship of medicine.

I know these are harsh words, but they need to be said. Have we forgotten the lessons learned a few centuries ago with scurvy, pernicious anaemia and pellagra? These horrendously deadly metabolic diseases were prevented by correcting a nutritional deficiency with a simple vitamin. What about the Pakistani Hunzakuts, some still fathering children at 110 years of age, surviving in many cases to great ages with no trace of cancer in their tribe? In comparison, let us take an honest look at our modern First World hospitals packed with desperately sick cancer sufferers, the latest in hi-tech gadgets, wise practitioners, $200-a-month health plans and a cancer slaughter rate that is now

---

[64] Day, Phillip & Steven Ransom, *World Without AIDS*, ibid.

claiming victims in one in every third family across the western world. And isn't it comforting to know that all this is presided over by the American Cancer Society, the world's wealthiest 'non-profit' institution[65] and the only known 'charity' that makes political contributions?

We mentioned earlier that the world still hosts cultures who are cancer-free. Tribes like the Abkhasians, the Azerbaijanis, the Hunzas, the Eskimaux and the Karakorum all live on nitriloside-rich food[66] and report not a single recognised case of cancer during the extended periods they have been studied by western gerontologists.

I was interviewed by radio station KFM in Tonbridge, England. The news reporter who did the interview was from the Karakorum tribe of Pakistan. She could verify that her people lived in many cases to great ages because of their diet. Their food is taken variously from buckwheat, peas, broad beans, lucerne, turnips, lettuce, sprouting pulse or gram, apricots with their seeds and berries of various kinds[67]. Their diet can be carrying as much as 250–3,000mg of B17 nitriloside in a daily ration. The average western diet contains less than 2mg of nitriloside a day. Interestingly, natives of these tribes, who move into urban, 'civilised' areas and change their diets accordingly, always begin to fall foul of cancer at the regular western incidence[68].

Krebs reports, concerning his studies into the dietary habits of these tribes: *"Upon investigating the diet of these people, we found that the seed of the apricot was prized as a delicacy and that every part of the apricot was utilized. We found that the major source of fats used for cooking was the apricot seed, and that the apricot oil*

---

[65] **Epstein, Dr Samuel** "American Cancer Society Indicted by the Cancer Prevention Coalition for Losing the Winnable War Against Cancer", www.preventcancer.com

[66] Foods rich in Vitamin B17.

[67] All these foods, with the exception of lettuce and turnips, contain high quantities of nitriloside.

[68] **Stefansson, Vilhjalmur** CANCER: Disease of Civilisation? An Anthropological and Historical Study, Hill & Wang, New York, 1960.

71

was so produced as inadvertently to admit a fair concentration of nitriloside or traces of cyanide into it[69]."

Western gerontologists have long studied such tribes in order to isolate the factors that appear to keep them free of degenerative diseases. Nobel laureate Dr Albert Schweitzer remarked in 1913:

"On my arrival in Gabon, I was astonished to encounter no case of cancer[70]."

Dr Stanislas Tancho, addressing the Academy of Sciences in 1843, repeated the remarks of a Doctor Bac, working as surgeon-in-chief of the Second African Regiment, who failed to come across even one case of cancer in Senegal. The surgeon-in-chief at Val-de-Grace in Algiers, a M. Baudens, was also mentioned by Dr Tancho. Baudens had worked for eight years in Algiers, coming across only two cases of cancer[71].

Concerning the Thlinget Eskimos of Alaska, the Reverend Livingston French Jones wrote in 1914:

"While certain diseases have always been found among the Thlingets, others that now afflict them are of recent introduction. Tumours, cancers and toothache were unknown to them until within recent years[72]."

Dr Samuel King Hutton remarked: *"Some diseases common in Europe have not come under my notice during a prolonged and careful survey of the health of the [Labrador] Eskimos. Of these diseases, the most striking is cancer[73]."*

---

[69] **Krebs, Ernst T** *Nutritional and Therapeutic Implications*, John Beard Memorial Foundation (privately published), 1964

[70] **Berglas, Alexander** Preface to *Cancer: Nature, Cause and Cure,* Paris, 1957

[71] **Tancho, Dr Stanislas** *Memoir on the Frequency of Cancer* (1843), quoted by Stefansson

[72] **Jones, Rev Livingston French** *A Study of the Thlingets of Alaska*, New York, 1914

[73] **Hutton, Dr Samuel King** *Among the Eskimos of Labrador,* London and Philadelphia 1912

Remarking on his interview with Joseph Herman Romig, dubbed 'Alaska's most famous doctor', Dr Preston A Price claims that *"...in his* [Romig's] *thirty-six years of contact with these people, he had never seen a case of malignant disease among the truly primitive Eskimos and Indians, although it frequently occurs when they are modernized[74]."*

These stories seem to be the same wherever non-westernised tribes are encountered. Lack of degenerative diseases in these indigenous tribes led famous explorer Roald Amundsen to comment in 1908:

"My sincerest wishes for our friends the Nechilli Eskimos is, that civilization may never reach them[75]."

The *Ecologist* magazine reports:

"Sir Robert McCarrison, a surgeon in the Indian Health Service, observed "a total absence of all diseases during the time I spent in the Hunza valley [seven years]... *During the period of my association with these peoples, I never saw a case of... cancer[76]."*

Dr Alexander Berglas sums up his own findings:

"Civilization is, in terms of cancer, a juggernaut that cannot be stopped... It is the nature and essence of industrial civilization to be toxic in every sense... We are faced with the grim prospect that the advance of cancer and of civilization parallel each other[77]."

Berglas' findings were of course to be corroborated by the World Health Organisation GNP/cancer incidence statistics we looked at earlier. The common denominator in each of the above cases contributing to a cancer-free society was a lack of toxic,

---

[74] **Price, Dr Weston A** *Nutrition and Physical Degeneration*, London and New York, 1939

[75] **Amundsen, Roald** *The Northwest Passage*, London and New York, 1908

[76] *The Ecologist,* Vol. 28, No. 2, March/April 1998, p. 95

[77] Berglas, Dr Alexander, ibid.

industrialised environment and a natural diet rich in minerals and the nitrilosides.

The other main factor influencing many of the health disasters afflicting the West today centres around our rabid consumption of meat and the way we culturally combine proteins and carbohydrates. As we learned earlier, according to research[78], a diet rich in animal proteins robs our body of its vital supplies of pancreatic enzymes, which are used by the body to terminate healing processes once they are completed[79]. These enzymes are employed during the complicated process the body undergoes as these foreign proteins are broken down into their constituent amino acids and reconstructed as human proteins – a process that is extremely taxing on the body's resources.

Our society has bought into the fear of dying through lack of protein, most believing that unless we scarf down meats by the rack-load, we are in serious danger of becoming protein-deficient. This dangerous nonsense came from initial trials conducted on rats. Later it was determined that rats require up to ten times more protein than humans, as evidenced by the commensurate increase in rat mothers' proteins in milk as compared with the protein content of human milk. Today, it is recognised that human protein requirements are not nearly as great as formerly assumed. Nevertheless, the protein-scoffing trend has been hard to exorcise from the minds of the laity, which in turn has led to an overabundance of illnesses and scourges in the West, as Dr Ethel Nelson points out:

"Some of today's most prevalent and devastating diseases in the United States have now been credited to excessive consumption of meat and animal products (milk, cheese, eggs, etc.) and insufficient ingestion of plant foods. These conditions include the so-called "Western diseases": coronary heart disease, diabetes, obesity, appendicitis, diverticulosis of the colon, hiatus

---

[78] *Cancer Control Journal,* Vol. 6. No.1-6
[79] Binzel MD, Philip, ibid.

hernia, hemorrhoids, varicose veins, cancer, osteoporosis, kidney disorders and accelerated sexual development in children.[80]

These diseases, relatively rare in the 1930s, are now found in ever increasing abundance among the 'well-fed' populations of the West. But research shows that ancient populations were also cursed with the diseases that came from heavy meat consumption. In Exodus 15:26 of the Bible, we read:

"If you diligently heed the voice of the Lord your God and do what is right in His sight, give ear to His commandments and keep all His statutes, I will put none of the diseases on you which I have brought on the Egyptians."

What were these diseases of the Egyptians? For that answer, we go to Dr Marc Armand Ruffer, a paleopathologist who, along with his associates, has performed over 36,000 autopsies on Egyptian mummified remains of Pharaonic royals. Ruffer's research demonstrates that most of the diseases striking the Egyptian royalty bear an uncanny resemblance to those killing us today: atherosclerosis (hardening of the arteries), heart disease, cancer, osteoporosis, obesity, tooth decay, arthritis, diverticulosis of the colon, and early sexual development in children. That these diseases were, in the main, being caused by excessive meat eating and wayward diets could be concluded by examining the presumably well-fed royal bodies to find cholesterol deposits with narrowing of the artery lumens.[81]

In 1992, heart disease alone was claiming 3,000 Americans *a day*. Colon and rectal cancers, now the second cause of cancer death in America, for years have been associated with high-animal-fat, low-fibre diets. Excessive bile acids are required to process high animal fats in the bowel and bile acids are carcinogenic to

---

[80] **Nelson MD, Ethel** *The Eden Diet and Modern Nutritional Research*, Twin Cities Conference 1992, Northwestern College, MN, USA.
[81] *Mysteries of the Mummies*, Loma Linda: Slide-tape program produced by Loma Linda University School of Health, 1984

humans.[82] The transit time for foods through the alimentary tract is prolonged with low-fibre bowel content, allowing a longer period of time for bile acids to act on bowel mucosa. High pork, beef and chicken consumption correlates closely with the incidence of colon cancer.[83]

Interestingly, Americans have two and a half times the incidence of colon cancer deaths as the Chinese, and yet Chinese-American women who adopt the high-fat, high-meat dietary habits of the United States suffer *four times* the rate of colon cancer as their counterparts in China. In Chinese-American males, the colorectal cancer rate is *seven times* that of their Chinese counterparts. Colon and rectal cancers increase more than 400% among sedentary people, which also correlates with the increased incidence of constipation in this group.[84]

High animal-fat diets have also been linked to breast cancer since high estrogen levels are a predominant factor in breast cancers. Meat-eating women have higher levels of estrogen in the urine than vegetarian women, according to research.[85]

All of which goes to show that there are some serious problems with Western diets that are still not being addressed. Heart disease and cancer, described by experts as being *preventable*, are the two leading killers in the Western world today.

Digestion is the single most strenuous activity our bodies undergo, which is why, after one of our cultural 'heart-attack-on-a-plate' breakfasts, we feel like we are walking on the surface of

[82] **Galloway, D** *Experimental colorectal cancer: The relationship of diet and faecal bile acid concentration to tumour induction.* Br. J. Surg. 73:233-237, 1986

[83] **Berg, J** Quoted in **Robbins, J** *Diet for a New America*, Stillpoint Publ. 1987. p.254

[84] **Whittemore, A** *Diet, physical activity and colorectal cancer among Chinese in North America and China*, J Natl. Cancer Inst. 82:915-926, 1990. Also Nelson MD, Ethel, ibid.

[85] **Schultz, T** *Nutrient intake and hormonal status of premenopausal vegetarian Seventh Day Adventist and premenopausal non-vegetarians. Nutr. Cancer* 4:247-259, 1983

Jupiter and beg God to take us from the knee down. Excessive meat consumption, coupled with bad food combining of proteins and starches, is also the reason why man is the only creature on Earth that has to process its food using medication – antacids! Other creatures do not improperly combine their foods. As Harvey Diamond, author of *Fit For Life*, wryly remarks, you almost never see a lion eating a zebra along with a baked potato.

But pick up any menu in a Western restaurant today, and you will see that the majority of items on offer in the starter and entrée sections consist of improperly combined proteins and carbohydrates – and mostly cooked to destroy many of the nutrients. Steak and fries, chicken and pasta, eggs on toast... the list of woes is as endless as the problems these combinations cause. Because the body produces acids to digest proteins and alkalis for carbohydrates, the two types of juices neutralise each other, eventually producing a rotting mass, parts of which in some cases can still be putrefying inside us up to 70 hours later! This digestive gridlock produces toxic by-products that get filed around the body and will stay in our systems until we detoxify – which again we almost never do as this is culturally not practised in our society today. On the other hand, proper food combining avoids this build-up and assists in detoxifying our systems from food abuse.

The full science of Natural Hygiene is a fascinating and satisfying study for each of us to make, but unfortunately beyond the scope of this book. One word on properly consuming fruit however. It has been found that the body's elimination (detoxification) cycle runs from approximately 4am to 12 noon in a normal, clock-adjusted body. This is the reason why we awaken with 'fur' on our tongues, bear's breath on the sheets (hhhhello, honey!) and a desire to go to the bathroom that won't quit. This is our body's time for shedding unwanted weight, ridding the system of toxic by-products and getting the human re-booted for the coming day.

But what do we do to disrupt this natural cycle? Four stacks of Aunt Lily's Arkansas pancakes and syrup go down the hatch during our cultural breakfast (the one we tell everyone we can't do without), or the British variation which is something like: two fried eggs, toast, sausages, bacon, tomatoes, washed down with coffee, followed up by a cigarette or two and the *Sun* newspaper.

More toxic gridlock results. But the worse thing is, the body is prevented from allocating its resources to shedding weight and cleaning itself out, which is essentially the same as detoxifying all the gunk that later gets layered onto the insides of our colons and elsewhere around our bodies. Other methods the body can use to get stuff out of the system are similarly compromised by our culture, like for instance our habit of firing aluminium-laced anti-perspirants directly into our lymph nodes, jamming them up with an element that has long been linked to the raging incidence of Alzheimer's Disease. Then we scrape the fur off our tongues using toothpastes laced with the main constituent of rat poison (sodium fluoride) and rinse our mouths out with water containing chlorine and highly toxic hexafluorosilicic acid, the 'fluoride' with which our governments contaminate our water supplies, which is the toxic waste product taken from phosphate fertilizer pollution scrubbers. Are you beginning to understand the *real* mess our bodies are in?

Fruit is an ideal way to detoxify the gunk in our systems during the morning elimination cycle. Ignore your fat grannies when they tell you not to eat too much fruit or the world will fall out of your tail-pipe. Your fat grannies are telling you this because their fat mommas told them the same thing. A fat person is simply someone who has not allowed his or her body to detoxify. Yes, overweight and obesity generally arise as a result of what we have put into our bodies, but our continued overweight and unhealthy condition exists because we are not allowing our system to take out the garbage because we jam up our bodies further with our cultural peccadilloes, like the big breakfast.

Ideally fruit should always be consumed ALONE ON AN EMPTY STOMACH. *Ideally too, the only thing you should consume from the time you arise to lunch-time should be fruit.* Try an experiment for a month and toss out the big breakfast in favour of eating nothing but pieces of fruit in the mornings. The panic clouding your features at this moment at the thought of having to go without the usual breakfast bulk will be off-set with the pleasurable knowledge that your hunger pangs will soon depart once your blood sugar levels regulate your cravings. If it helps, promise yourself the usual heart-attack-on-a-plate if you do not feel satisfied thirty minutes after eating all the fruit you wish to eat. Pineapple, grapes, peaches, oranges, apples, pears (of course, eat the seeds too where appropriate) are all the best kit to get into the kitchen for this great little experiment.

Then when you get to lunch, have lunch! But combine proteins with high water-content vegetables or salad, not with pasta, potatoes, or similar. CUT WAY DOWN ON THE ANIMAL MEAT. Vegetables and salad ideally should be enjoyed as close to their native forms (raw and unadulterated) as you can manage. Organic produce is best, uncontaminated with pesticides and other problems we will examine a little later.

Three things will start to happen almost immediately you commence this regimen: firstly, the world will fall out of your tail-pipe. This is your body finally beginning to send the garbage packing. It's all a bit of a mess, but it's leaving – and that's the good news. Loose stools produced from this eating regimen are by no means unhealthy and should be encouraged with as much fruit (on an empty stomach in the morning) and high water-content veggies (later in the day) as you can manage. Secondly, You will begin to experience a satisfying return of energy and well-being. Thirdly, you will experience a rapid, satisfying and steady weight-loss as you proceed with eating your food the way the body likes to process it.

Regular stool-passing is a sign that everything is on the move again. No more 'troubled interactions with nourishment', as the psychologists delightfully put it. A new 'you' is emerging as you detoxify. Your skin will appear fresher and healthier looking, your eyes will look clearer, you will sleep better, you will walk funny for a few weeks until the loose stools firm up again, but MOST IMPORTANTLY, your body has been given back its driver's licence and is now in the hot-seat correctly processing the body's tasks when it should, how it should and why it should.

After four weeks of this experiment, go back and try to eat the heart-attack-on-a-plate for breakfast. You will feel like you have just swallowed the state of Montana, mountains 'n all. And you won't want to do it again.

Creating your own toxin-free environment too begins and ends with INDIVIDUAL common sense. As Mr Industry, Mrs Corporate Drug-Healthcare and Nanny Government are not likely ride in to rescue us any time soon, you, Mrs Smith... you, Mr Williams... you, young Robert... and you, grandma, are going to have to do it for yourselves. Because the food supplies these days are largely depleted of their natural mineral content, supplementation of highly absorbable vitamins, minerals and antioxidants needs to happen in your household, and we're going to come back to this important subject a little later on.

But as we have seen, diets need to change immediately. Suppliers of organically grown fruits and vegetables need to be ferreted out and used henceforth, albeit at greater expense, as our primary food source. There's another irony in this whole bag of potatoes. Natural food is costing more because it isn't pumped full of preservatives and so doesn't last as long in the stores. But, as you will discover, a messy miracle starts to happen when you eat good, clean and wholesome, high-water-content fruits and veggies AND CUT WAY DOWN ON THE MEAT AND OTHER ANIMAL PROTEINS (do you think I have emphasised this enough yet?!). Your body will begin detoxifying the garbage and dropping needless weight at a splendid rate and you feel the benefits of it almost immediately.

I want you to obtain a copy of Harvey and Marilyn Diamond's excellent bestseller *Fit For Life – Part 1* for a fuller treatment on this great subject of Natural Hygiene[86]. I cannot recommend a book

---

[86] **Diamond, Harvey & Marilyn** *Fit For Life – Parts 1 & 2*, Little, Brown & Company, 1987, ISBN 0446300152. Available through Credence Publications.

more highly than this one for well-grounded common sense when it comes to detoxifying your system and getting back to eating basics. This book is not about some magic new special diet. The authors concentrate on a natural, Hunza-like approach to putting the right gas back in your machine and have deservedly sold millions of copies to those who have decided to stop eating the plastic and the road-kill and re-take control of their own nutrition and healthcare. It will explain more about the simple Natural Hygiene program, the pitfalls of what has happened to our diets and how immediately we can start to put things right. I believe this book has already saved countless tens of thousands of lives. It could save yours too. And even better - it is a howling, hilarious read!

It is interesting and poignant to note that the observations outlined in this chapter were encountered over 50 years ago and yet today, modern cancer research still refuses to make nutrition and ecological toxicity a firm priority. As we will discover in the next chapter, this has been mostly due to the uncompromising conflicts of interest existing within the Medical/Industrial Complex which produces such chemical toxins to incredible profit[87].

---

[87] For in-depth information regarding the chemical industry's self-regulatory problems, see *The Ecologist*, Vol. 28, No. 2, March/April, 1998, p. 57-61. Also **Hall, Ross Hume** *Health and the Global Environment*, Polity Press, 1990

Living With the Chemistry Set
Environmental Contributions to Cancer

Norine Warnock lives downwind of the British Petroleum refinery and chemical plant located in Lima, Ohio:

"I have health problems and my four-year-old daughter has serious respiratory problems. Maybe those problems are not connected to BP, but maybe they are.... The guy across the street has cancer. The woman down the street has brain cancer. The woman around the corner has brain cancer. The woman who lives next door to my child's friend has cancer. The woman on the next block has breast cancer. The guy next door to her has cancer. And so does the woman next door to him. Those are just the houses I can see when I am looking out of my own front door[88]."

* * * * *

20th century civilised society manufactures and uses tens of thousands of new chemical substances every decade. From potent synergised pyrethrins in fly spray through petro-chemical oils in soaps and gasolines across to plastics in cars and additives in foods to keep them fresher in our supermarkets for longer periods of time, societies – indeed, the new global community, as the world is now renamed – use most of these products on a daily basis. These man-made substances do not naturally exist in nature, and so, as each new product and its chemistry presents itself as a new experience for mankind's own biology, common sense would dictate that stringent tests would be in place to ensure that the substance in question can be cleared for safe usage.

Agencies, such as Britain's Environment Agency and America's Environmental Protection Agency (EPA) exist, so far as the public is concerned, for no other reason than to ensure that we can raise our families and work at our jobs in, as far as possible, a contamination-free environment. All technologically advanced

---

[88] *The Ecologist,* Vol. 28, ibid.

nations have such environmental agencies, and yet every year, people still die by the hundreds of thousands, polluted and poisoned by these substances. So what has gone so very wrong?

The major problem stems from the rate at which new chemicals and chemical products are pouring onto the world's markets. Government agencies, already so tightly controlled financially with annual budget constraints, simply do not have the resources to test everything. Therefore they must rely heavily on industry-sponsored reports on product safety *from the manufacturers themselves*, which naturally opens up a wide arena for abuse. Agencies such as the EPA threaten dire fines on pharmaceutical and chemical companies found indulging in any foul play in order to ram potentially unsafe products through regulation. But prosecution of such cases by government on a realistic scale is rare since litigation consumes prodigious amounts of taxpayers' money.

This dangerous, if intriguing problem has provoked an angry backlash from 'green-minded' citizens and has led to the formation of other more independent watchdogs, who in turn write their own reports. America's Center for Public Integrity (CPI) recently issued a report appropriately entitled: *Toxic Deception: How the Chemical Industry Manipulates Science, Bends the Law, and Endangers Your Health*. This slamming indictment on the world's Industrial/Chemical Complex was authored by *Newsday* reporter Dan Fagin and *National Law Journal's* Marianne Lavelle. The bottom line of the report's conclusion confirmed what was already known: that the chemical industry was largely self-regulatory. But another more sinister dimension emerged. Namely, that safety studies performed by chemical industry sponsors tended to find chemicals innocent of health risks to the public while non-chemical researchers invariably found substantial risks associated with these same substances.

In the area of pesticides, Fagin's CPI report states that 90% of America's 1650 'weed' scientists rely heavily on grants from pesticide manufacturers. Usually these men and women are the very researchers running studies on new pesticides products for the government! These industry reports are taken seriously by the US government, which has largely adopted the line that a chemical is safe unless proven otherwise.

Russell Mokhiber, editor of *Corporate Crime Reporter* (Washington DC), has made a detailed study of the CPI report. He states:

"In 1991 and 1992, when the [US government's] Environmental Protection Agency offered amnesty from big-money fines to any manufacturer who turned in health studies that they should have provided under the law earlier, more than 10,000 studies suddenly appeared, showing that their products already on the market pose a substantial risk[89]."

The CPI report was highly critical of the EPA's efforts to police private laboratories that conduct important safety tests. The Center for Public Integrity's executive director Charles Lewis tells us: *"The EPA has never inspected about 1,550 of the 2,000 labs doing the manufacturer-funded studies that the EPA uses to decide whether chemicals are safe. The EPA, which does not do its own safety tests, has audited only about 3.5% of the hundreds of thousands of studies that have been submitted to the agency."*

CPI also discovered many revolving doors between the US government and the chemical industry. Of 344 lobbyists and lawyers who admitted to working within the chemical industry and trade associations between 1990 and 1995, at least 135 originally came from federal agencies or congressional offices. More than this, a substantial number of senior EPA officials working in toxics and pesticides for the government were later found to have left government employment to take up related positions within the chemical industry. Lewis remarks: *"There are many tales of former US officials helping the industry to thwart federal government oversight."*

---

[89] **Mokhiber, Russell** *"Objective" Science at Auction, The Ecologist,* Vol. 28, No.2, March/April 1998

Russell Mokhiber again: *"At least 3,363 trips were taken between March 1993 and March 1995 by EPA officials that were paid for – to the tune of $3 million – by corporations, universities, trade associations, environmental organizations and private sponsors.... Members of Congress have also been courted by chemical companies. The manufacturers of alachor, atrazine, formaldehyde and perchloroethylene provided 214 free trips to members of Congress and flew one key committee chairman to Rio de Janeiro[90]."*

The Toxic Substances Control Act was passed by Congress in 1976. The aim of this law was to decide which of the 70,000-plus substances in public use should be tested for toxicity. Once again, it must be stressed that even the United States federal government, with its limited funding in this area, has scant resources to conduct a large number of its own safety tests. In spite of this fact, the National Toxicology Program (NTP) was set up, involving eight federal agencies, specifically to test for carcinogenic properties of selected substances. The reality of the NTP is that only a few dozen target chemicals are tested each year in any detail. Researcher Peter Montague argues that even these tests are useless, since they do not examine the effects of these substances on the nervous system, the endocrine system, the immune system and on major organs, such as the heart, liver, lungs, kidney and brain. He writes:

"During a typical year, while the National Toxicology Program is studying the cancer effects of one or two dozen chemicals, about 1,000 new chemicals enter commercial markets. Our federal government is simply swamped by new chemicals and cannot keep up. Furthermore, it is highly unlikely that this situation will change. No one believes that our government – or anyone else – will ever have the capacity to evaluate fully the dangers of 1,000 new chemicals each year, especially not in combination with the 70,000 chemicals already in circulation[91]."

---

[90] Mokhiber, Russell, ibid.

[91] **Montague, Peter** edits the Environmental Research Foundation's weekly publication, *Rachel's Environment and Health Weekly*, PO Box 5036, Annapolis, MD 21403-70336 USA

And if the EPA gets cute with any of the major chemical corporations, Montague continues, lawyers acting for the chemical industry know they can tie up the EPA in long and expensive legal snarls for decades. The idea that government can regulate big business is ridiculous, he concludes. *"We could multiply the size of our federal government by ten (a truly frightening thought), and it would still be no match for the Fortune 500."*

Most who have studied the situation in some detail have concluded that a health disaster of monumental proportions will probably be the only way to compel a strategic change in public thinking. The chemical industry will never gain an instant morality. Ross Hume Hall makes this comment:

"We find ourselves in a similar position to that of our nineteenth century forebears. The major health issue then was infectious disease. They had no cure for typhoid or cholera, but instead launched vast public health programs of clean water, uncontaminated food and better living conditions, which eliminated much of the disease then burdening 19th century society. Such programs proved that human suffering due to illness and premature death, not to mention the medical-care costs, can be reduced or eliminated by effective social policy[92]."

Standing in the dawn of this new millennium, our world faces an unprecedented crisis with its environment. Diseases that were all but unknown before the Industrial Revolution are now marching in step with our rapacious delight in stretching the control-bounds of our biotechnology. Cancer, multiple sclerosis, AIDS, ME (chronic fatigue), Alzheimers, diabetes, Parkinsons, coronary heart disease are all illnesses familiar to us, striking down family and friends with such grim reality that few expect these days to die of 'natural causes'. But are we just the innocent bystanders?

---

[92] Hall, Ross Hume, ibid.

We fill our tooth cavities with mercury amalgam, a slow-release neurotoxic metal[93]. We cook our food in aluminium pots and pans and spray aluminium compounds directly into our lymph-nodes. We drink sugar-laced sodas from aluminium cans in scant disregard of the connections aluminium has with Alzheimer's Disease. We allow our drinking water to be laced with chlorine and highly dangerous hexafluorosilicic acid, toxic industry waste (this substance is generically referred to as 'fluoride'). The very food we eat has become corrupted by organophosphates, permeated with pesticides, stripped of minerals and now is increasingly genetically modified.

The average apple sold off the supermarket shelf we will have saturated with chlorpyrifos, captan, iprodione, vinclozolin and then sealed in wax for longer shelf life. These pesticides, when tested, have variously caused birth defects, cancer, impaired immune response, fungal growth, genetic damage and disruption to the endocrine system. The average vitamin-depleted white bread roll can be tested positive for pesticides such as chlorpyrifos-methyl, endosulfasulphate, chlorothalonil, dothiocarbamates, iprodione, procymidone and vinclozolin[94].

Whilst living in Southern California, I witnessed the population of the Southland being routinely sprayed with malathion from helicopters originating from a covert government base at Evergreen, Arizona. Malathion is an organophosphate which can cause gene and immune system damage, behavioural deficits in newborns and small children, is a suspect viral enhancer and implicated in Reye's Syndrome. The purpose of the spraying is to kill the Mediterranean fruit fly which, for some 'inexplicable' reason, prefers the concrete jungle of Los Angeles, East LA and South Pasadena to its indigenous habitat among the orchards and green pastures of central California to the north. The malathion warnings would go out over the radio: *"Cover up your cars and take your pets indoors, folks. But don't worry, it won't hurt you."*

---

[93] Some Mexico cancer clinics, such as the Oasis Hospital, commence a patient's laetrile cancer therapy by first removing all mercury amalgam fillings and replacing them with non-toxic substitutes.
[94] *The New Zealand Total Diet Survey*, 1990/1

"Milk – It Does a Body Good". Who are we kidding with what is fed to the average cow today (including steroids, antibiotics, human sewage and food fillers such as sawdust, concrete dust and paper)? Beef, pork, chicken and lamb read like a *Who's Who* of mankind's latest bold advances in steroid-bolstered, hormone-accelerated quota production. If we are what we eat, then man is indeed taking a quantum step in DEvolution. As my fellow researcher Wendy Wallace astutely points out, maybe we ARE devolving... devolving back into pond scum whence we supposedly came, and our minds are so far along in the process, we just can't figure it out.

The majority of illnesses striking us today are metabolic and toxin-related in origin, which our establishment attempts to combat with the drugs and chemicals it has been trained to research and dispense. But metabolic diseases, as we will learn, can only be successfully regressed with metabolic preventatives, or food factors, which themselves provide the establishment with scant opportunity for profit, since they cannot be proprietarily owned or patented. Worse, the very government regulatory agencies themselves, such as the US Food & Drug Administration and Britain's Medicines Control Agency (MCA), which are supposed to protect the public from potentially dangerous products coming onto the market, are horribly compromised because of personal investments or ties with the chemical/drug industries. A USA TODAY analysis of financial conflicts at 159 FDA advisory committee meetings from 1st January to 30th June 2000 finds that:

- At 92% of the meetings, at least one member had a financial conflict of interest.
- At 55% of meetings, half or more of the FDA advisers had conflicts of interest.
- Conflicts were most frequent at the 57 meetings when broader issues were discussed: 92% of members had conflicts.

- At the 102 meetings dealing with the fate of a specific drug, 33% of the experts had a financial conflict.[95]

"The best experts for the FDA are often the best experts to consult with industry," says FDA senior associate commissioner Linda Suydam, who is in charge of waiving conflict-of-interest restrictions. But Larry Sasich of Public Citizen, an advocacy group, says, *"The industry has more influence on the process than people realize."*

Britain's Medicines Control Agency fares little better with its track record for impartiality when it comes to regulating the drug industry. According to a Daily Express investigation, key members of the Committee on Safety of Medicines and the Medicines Commission themselves have heavy personal investments in the drug industry. Yet these committees are the ones which decide which drugs are allowed onto the market and which are rejected!

According to the report, two thirds of the 248 experts sitting on the Medicines Commission have financial ties to the pharmaceutical industry. Drug regulators such as Dr Richard Auty have £110,000 worth of holdings with AstraZeneca. Dr Michael Denham owns £115,000 worth of shares in SmithKline Beecham. Dr Richard Logan has up to £30,000 shares in AstraZeneca, SmithKline Beecham and Glaxo Wellcome. Logan's role with the committee involves examining cases where a drug might have to be withdrawn from the market for safety reasons.

David Ganderton was an advisor for nine years with the CSM panel who used to work for AstraZeneca. His current shareholding with this drug company is worth £91,000. Other members of the committees with substantial holdings for example include Dr Colin Forfar, with £22,000 with Glaxo Wellcome and Dr Brian Evans owning £28,000 worth of shares with Glaxo Wellcome.[96]

---

[95] *USA Today* article by Dennis Cauchon, *FDA Advisers Tied to Industry*, 25th September 2000, http://www.usatoday.com/news/washdc/ncssun06.htm

[96] *Daily Express* micro edition, 6th August 2000

The Daily Express report goes on to tell us: *"Tom Moore, a former senior executive with AstraZeneca, told the Sunday Express that the drug companies go out of their way to build strong links. He said, "Their objective is to get as close as possible. They are an extremely powerful lobby group because they have unlimited resources."*

The [drug] *companies provide* [members of CSM and other regulatory committees] *trips abroad to conferences, large research grants that can keep a university department employed for years, and consultancies that can boost an academic's humble income."*

On the other hand, it is quite easy to understand why nutritional treatments and preventative medicine pose such a threat to this massively funded industry surrounding sickness and why they are almost never used as the primary therapy. One drug alone can cost over $200 million to go through regulation in America. Who is ever going to recoup such a cost with a vitamin or herbal treatment that cannot be patented? And herein lies the problem deadlocking western healthcare's ability to halt Western diseases. Most of these diseases killing us are metabolic- or toxin-related and by their very definition cannot be treated with drugs or other proprietary therapies such as radiation. Yet patented treatments form the bulwark of Western medicine's tremendous wealth and power! This is the reason why western healthcare is conspicuously failing to halt killers such as heart disease or cancer. The real remedies and preventatives have no commercial value.

Now we are in a position to see clearly why isolated tribes like the Hunzas, living in a non-industrialised environment, breathing pollution-free air, drinking chemical-free water, exercising regularly and eating wholesome fruits and vegetables rich in minerals and B17 nitrilosides, can remain free of the degenerative illnesses that are literally killing the 'civilised' human race all around them. There's a major parable in there somewhere, isn't there? So what can we do? How can we be more Hunza-like in our approach to our food and environment?

A Rat Control Program?

Most people have no idea what the personal care products they use every day are doing to them. As an example, in 1990, 38,000 cosmetic injuries were reported in the US that required medical attention[97]. Health concerns are continuously being raised about ingredients in shampoos, toothpastes, skin creams, and other personal care products. In fact, researchers in Japan, Germany, Switzerland, and the US say many ingredients in personal care products may be related to premature baldness, cataract formation, environmental cancers, contact dermatitis and possible eye damage in young children. We'll find out what some of these substances actually are in a moment and why these researchers have every reason to be concerned.

The National Institute of Occupational Safety and Health has found that 884 chemicals available for use in cosmetics have been reported to the US Government as toxic substances[98]. So why are these potentially harmful ingredients allowed in personal care products?

In 1938 the US Government created a legal definition for cosmetics by passing The Federal Food, Drug and Cosmetic Act. Cosmetics were defined as products for *"cleansing, beautifying, promoting attractiveness, or altering the appearance."* In this definition, a cosmetic is defined *"in terms of its intended purpose rather than in terms of the ingredients with which it is formulated."*[99] Although the Food and Drug Administration classifies cosmetics, incredibly it does not regulate them. According to a document posted on the agency's World Wide Web homepage, *"a cosmetic*

---

[97] **Steinman, D & Samuel S Epstein** *The Safe Shopper's Bible*, pp. 182-183, ISBN 0020820852; also Consumer Product Safety Commission (CPSC), Product summary report: Washington DC, 1990

[98] Steinman, D & S Epstein, *Safe Shopper's Bible*, ibid.

[99] Consumer Health and Product Hazards/Cosmetic Drugs, Pesticides, Food Additives, Volume 2 of The Legislation of Product Safety, edited by Samuel S Epstein and Richard D Grundy, MIT Press, 1974

manufacturer may use any ingredient or raw material and market the final products without government approval[100]."

On 10th September 1997, Senator Edward M. Kennedy of Massachusetts, while discussing the FDA reform bill, stated, *"The cosmetic industry has borrowed a page from the playbook of the tobacco industry, by putting profits ahead of public health."* Kennedy further stated, *"Cosmetics can be dangerous to your health. Yet this greedy industry wants Congress to prevent the American people from learning that truth. Every woman who uses face cream, or hair spray, or lipstick, or shampoo, or mascara, or powder should demand that this arrogant and irresponsible power-play by the industry be rejected. A study by the respected, non-partisan General Accounting Office reported that more than 125 ingredients available for use in cosmetics are suspected of causing cancer. Other cosmetics may cause adverse effects on the nervous system, including convulsions. Still other ingredients are suspected of causing birth defects. A carefully controlled study found that one in sixty users suffered a cosmetic related injury identified by a physician[101]."*

In 1998 Peter Phillips and *Project Censored* listed the year's top 25 censored stories. The number 2 censored story (as detailed in his book) was titled "Personal Care and Cosmetic Products May Be Carcinogenic[102]."

Shocking news indeed. Let's take a brief look at a few of the ingredients that top the list of potentially harmful compounds that are present in products we use every day.

Sodium Lauryl Sulfate (SLS)
SLS is a very harsh detergent found in almost all shampoos and more than a few toothpastes. Pick up a cross-section of these

---

[100] http://vm.cfsan.fda.gov/~dms/cos-hdb1.html
[101] This statement is quoted from Senator Kennedy's office on http://www.senate.gov/~kennedy/statements /970910fda.html
[102] **Phillips, Peter** *Censored 1998: The News That Didn't Make the News*, Project Censored, 1998 ISBN 1888363649

products next time you visit the supermarket and you will find SLS or SLES in pride of place under the ingredients label. SLS started its career as an industrial degreasant and garage floor cleaner. When applied to human skin it has the effect of stripping off the oil layer and then irritating and eroding the skin, leaving it rough and pitted. Studies[103] have shown that:

- Shampoos with SLS could retard healing and keep children's eyes from developing properly. Children under six years old are especially vulnerable to improper eye development (Summary of Report of Research to Prevent Blindness, Inc. conference)
- SLS can cause cataracts in adults and delays the healing of wounds in the surface of the cornea.
- SLS has a low molecular weight and so is easily absorbed by the body. It builds up in the heart, liver, lungs and brain and can cause major problems in these areas.
- SLS causes skin to flake and to separate and causes substantial roughness on the skin.
- SLS causes dysfunction of the biological systems of the skin
- SLS is such a caustic cleanser that it actually corrodes the hair follicle and impairs its ability to grow hair.
- SLS is routinely used in clinical studies to deliberately irritate the skin so that the effects of other substances can be tested[104].

Ethoxylation
Ethoxylation is the process that makes degreasing agents such as sodium lauryl sulfate (SLS) less abrasive and gives them enhanced foaming properties. When SLS is ethoxylated, it forms sodium laureth sulfate (SLES), a compound used in many shampoos, toothpastes, bath gels, bubble baths, and industrial degreasants. The problem is, the extremely harmful compound 1,4-dioxane may be created during the ethoxylation process. 1,4-dioxane was one of the principal components of the chemical defoliant Agent Orange, used to great effect during the Vietnam

---

[103] **Vance, Judi** *Beauty to Die For*, Promotion Publishing, 1998 ISBN 1576010350
[104] Study cited by *The Wall Street Journal*, 1st November 1988

War to strip off the jungle canopy to reveal the enemy. 1,4-dioxane is a hormonal disrupter believed to be the chief agent implicated in the host of cancers suffered by Vietnam military personnel after the war. It is also an estrogen mimic thought to increase the chances of breast and endometrial cancers, stress-related illnesses and lower sperm counts.

Leading toxicologist Dr Samuel Epstein reports: *"The best way to protect yourself is to recognize ingredients most likely to be contaminated with 1,4-dioxane. These include ingredients with the prefix word, or syllable PEG, Polyethylene, Polyethylene Glycol, Polyoxyethylene, eth (as in sodium laureth sulfate), or oxynol. Both polysorbate 60 and polysorbate 80 may also be contaminated with 1,4-dioxane[105]."*

Propylene Glycol

Propylene glycol is a common ingredient used extensively in industry as a component of brake fluids, paint, varnishes and anti-freeze compounds. It also appears in many beauty creams, cleansers, makeup and children's personal care products. Judi Vance writes: *"If you were to purchase a drum of this chemical from a manufacturer, he is required to furnish you with a material safety data sheet (MSDS) and it may alarm you to find that this common, widely used humectant has a cautionary warning in its MSDS that reads: "If on skin: thoroughly wash with soap and water."[90]*

The American Academy of Dermatologists published a clinical review in January 1991 that showed propylene glycol caused a significant number of reactions and was a primary irritant to the skin even in low levels of concentration (around 5%). However propylene glycol routinely appears in the top three ingredients of a given product, indicating that it is present in high concentration[106]. It has been shown that propylene glycol:

---

[105] Epstein, Dr Samuel *Safe Shopper's Bible,* p. 190-191

[106] The first two or three ingredients listed on a product label usually constitute over half of a formulation. In some products, the first two or three ingredients can constitute 70-90% of the formulation. Ingredients are listed in descending order,

- Has severe adverse health effects and has been found to cause kidney damage, and liver abnormalities.
- Damages cell membranes causing rashes, dry skin, contact dermatitis and surface damage to the skin.
- Is toxic to human cells in cultures.

Diethanolamine (DEA)
Cocamide DEA
Lauramide DEA

A colourless liquid or crystalline alcohol that is used as a solvent, emulsifier, and detergent (wetting agent). DEA works as an emollient in skin-softening lotions or as a humectant in other personal care products. When found in products containing nitrates, it reacts chemically with the nitrates to form potentially carcinogenic nitrosamines. Although earlier studies seemed to indicate that DEA itself was not a carcinogen, more recent studies show that DEA has the capacity unequivocally to cause cancer, even in formulations that exclude nitrates[107]. DEA may also irritate the skin and mucous membranes[108]. Other ethanolamines to watch out for are: triethanolamine (TEA) and monethanolamine (MEA)

Fluorides (Sodium Fluoride and Hexafluorosilicic Acid)

Fluorides used in the drinking water supplies are a toxic, non-biodegradable, environmental pollutant, officially classified as a contaminant by the US Environmental Protection Agency. Shocking though it may be to contemplate, the reality is, these chemicals are simply hazardous industrial waste - a by-product from the manufacture of phosphate fertilisers, gleaned from this industry's pollution scrubbers - which is largely disposed of in our

---

going down to 1% concentration. Below 1%, ingredients may be listed in any order.

[107] **Epstein, Samuel S** *The Politics of Cancer Revisited*, East Ridge Press, 1998. p.479

[108] Many nitrosamines have been determined to cause cancer in laboratory animals. Nitrosamine contamination of cosmetics became an issue in early 1977. The Food & Drug Administration expressed its concern about the contamination of cosmetics in a Federal Register notice dated 10th April 1979, which stated that cosmetics containing nitrosamines may be considered adulterated and subject to enforcement action.

public water supply. Hexafluorosilicic acid, the most commonly used fluoridation additive, contains other toxic substances including lead, beryllium, mercury, cadmium, arsenic, and radionuceides[109]. Fluoride's beastliness was summed up in a terse statement issued by Dr Dean Burk of the National Cancer Institute: *"Fluoride causes more human cancer death, and causes it faster than any other chemical."* [110]

Fluorine is an extremely volatile, electronegative element that is never found alone in nature, and thus compounds readily with many elements. Fluorines were used as battlefield gas in both world wars and sodium fluoride is routinely used as a constituent of rat poison. Sodium fluoride is also a hazardous by-product of the aluminium smelting and sugar industries, but as most know, is incredibly used in toothpastes in high concentrations, apparently to reduce cavities. *"Whether there is another rat control program underway has never been publicly discussed,"* states veteran commentator Eustace Mullins, in conclusion to all his research. [111]

As far back as October of 1944, the *Journal of the American Medical Association* published an editorial stating: *"... that the use of drinking water containing as little as 1.2 to 3 parts per million of fluoride will cause such developmental disturbances in bones as osteosclerosis, spondylosis, and osteoporosis, as well as goitre."* [112]

In May 1992, Dr William Marcus, the senior science advisor and chief toxicologist with the United States Environmental Protection Agency, was fired from his post after publicly disclosing his frank comments concerning mass medicating the public without its consent and the appalling hazards of fluorides. Marcus was concerned that the results of US Government studies on fluoride, completed in 1984 and a second in 1987, were kept from the

---

[109] **d'Raye, Tonita**, *The Facts About Fluoride*, PO Box 21075, Keizer, OR 97307 USA
[110] d'Raye, Tonita, ibid
[111] Mullins, Eustace, ibid
[112] *Journal of the American Medical Association*, "Health Damaging Effects of Fluoride", October 1944

American public. After a long fight, Dr Marcus was reinstated on 28th February 1995. *"If this were any other chemical but fluoride,"* Marcus commented, *"there would be a call for the immediate cessation of its use. It shows potential for great harm[113]."*

The Safe Water Foundation filed Freedom on Information Act requests and to obtain the results of these government studies. Dr John Yiamouyiannis (president of the Safe Water Foundation) said *"All tests came out positive[114]."* (establishing a fluoride-cancer link)

Dr John R Lee MD, who was chairman of the Environmental Health Committee of his local medical association in Marin County, California, went head-to-head with authorities on the fluoride issue. According to Dr Lee, the county had continually pushed water fluoridation on the local ballot until it passed by a slim margin of one per cent. Lee states: *"[Fluoride] is a toxic waste product of many types of industry; for instance, glass production, phosphate fertilizer production and many others. They would have no way to dispose of the tons of fluoride waste they produce unless they could find some use for it, so they made up this story about it being good for dental health. Then they can pass it through everyone's bodies and into the sewer[115]."*

Lee's comments on their own would be shocking and dismissive. The problem is, hundreds of specialists, doctors and biochemists have been saying the same thing for years. And sure enough, when the curtains were finally pulled back and the veil of secrecy lifted, federal research indeed discovered that fluoride caused cancer in humans and animals[116]. NCI's Dr Burk stated: *"It is concluded that artificial fluoridation appears to cause or induce about 20-30 excess cancer deaths for every 100,000 persons exposed per year after about 15-20 years[117]."* Yet incredibly to this day, not only is fluoridation of the water supply and toothpaste still

---

[113] d'Raye, Tonita, ibid
[114] http://www.whale.to/Dental/fluoride.html
[115] http://www.thewinds.org/archive/medical/fluoride01-98.html
[116] National Toxicology Program (NTP) 1990, National Cancer Institute, HHS Fluoride Report 2/91
[117] http://www.thewinds.org/archive/medical/fluoride01-98.html

permitted, US federal goals require mandatory fluoridation of the water supply in 75% of all US cities by the close of the year 2000![118]

- Fluoride accumulates in the body like lead, inflicting its damage over long periods of time.
- Fluoride is more toxic than lead, and just slightly less toxic than arsenic[119].
- Medical research shows that hip fractures are 20-40% higher in fluoridated communities[120].

The American Medical Association (AMA) issued a news release titled "Study Links Fluoride to Rare Bone Cancer" on 8th December 1993. This study also showed that hip fractures were 27% higher in women, and 41% higher in men in the fluoridated city featured in the tests. Hip fractures (potentially fatal to the elderly) are linked to fluoridated water[121].

Other harmful personal care ingredients can include:

Alcohol
A colourless, volatile, flammable liquid produced by the fermentation of yeast and carbohydrates. Alcohol is used frequently as a solvent and is also found in beverages and medicine. As an ingredient in ingestible products, alcohol may cause body tissues to be more vulnerable to carcinogens. Mouthwashes with an alcohol content of 25 percent or more have been implicated in mouth, tongue and throat cancers, according to a 1991 study released by the National Cancer Institute. Also a disturbing trend in accidental poisonings has been attributed to alcohol consumption from mouthwashes. After the NCI figures were published, Warner Lambert, manufacturers of the mouthwash

---

[118] d'Raye, Tonita, ibid
[119] Clinical Toxicology, 1984
[120] The John R Lee MD *Medical Letter*, February 1999
[121] *Journal of the American Medical Association*, (JAMA 3/8/95, 8/11-12/92, 7/25/91, 6/19/91, 7/25/90; *American Journal of Epidemiology*, 4/91; *American Journal of Public Health*, 7/90

Listerine (26.9% alcohol), announced a new version of their product with significantly less alcohol[122].

Alpha Hydroxy Acid (AHA)
An organic acid produced by anaerobic respiration. Skin care products containing AHA exfoliate not only destroy skin cells, but the skin's protective barrier as well. Long-term skin damage may result from its use.

Alumin(i)um
A metallic element used extensively in the manufacture of aircraft components, prosthetic devices, and as an ingredient in antiperspirants, antacids, and antiseptics. Aluminium has long been linked to Alzheimer's Disease, which is currently afflicting 1 in 2 persons over the age of 70. Use of aluminium pots and pans to cook food and the use of aluminium cans for soda, as well as the unnecessary cultural penchant for spraying aluminium directly into our lymph nodes as underarm antiperspirant all give grave causes for concern.

Animal Fat (Tallow)
A type of animal tissue made up of oily solids or semisolids that are water-insoluble esters of glycerol and fatty acids. Animal fats and lye are the chief ingredients in bar soap, a cleaning and emulsifying product that may act as a breeding ground for bacteria.

Bentonite
A porous clay that expands to many times its dry volume as it absorbs water. Bentonite is commonly found in many cosmetic foundations and may clog pores and suffocate the skin. Bentonite is used by fire fighters to suffocate forest fires by eliminating the oxygen available.

Butane
Aerosol propellant. Flammable and in high doses may be narcotic or cause asphyxiation.

---

[122] *Wall Street Journal*, 23rd April 1991 p.B1, Ron Winslow

Collagen

An insoluble fibrous protein that is too large to penetrate the skin. The collagen found in most skin care products is derived from animal carcasses and ground up chicken feet. This ingredient forms a layer of film that may suffocate the skin.

Dioxin (see also Ethoxylation and 1,4-Dioxane)

A potentially carcinogenic by-product that results from the process used to increase foam levels in cleansers such as shampoos, tooth pastes, etc., and to bleach paper at paper mills. Dioxin-treated containers (and some plastic bottles) sometimes transfer dioxins to the products themselves. It has been shown that dioxin's carcinogenicity is up to 500,000 times more potent than that of DDT[123].

Elastin of High-Molecular Weight

A protein similar to collagen that is the main component of elastic fibres. Elastin is also derived from animal sources. Its effect on the skin is similar to collagen.

Fluorocarbons

A colourless, non-flammable gas or liquid that can produce mild upper respiratory tract irritation. Fluorocarbons are commonly used as a propellant in hairsprays.

Formaldehyde

A toxic, colourless gas that is an irritant and a carcinogen. When combined with water, formaldehyde is used as a disinfectant, fixative, or preservative. Formaldehyde is found in many cosmetic products and conventional nail care systems.

Glycerin

A syrupy liquid that is chemically produced by combining water and fat. Glycerin is used as a solvent and plasticiser. Unless the humidity of air is over 65%, glycerin draws moisture from the lower

---

[123] Epstein, Dr Samuel *Safe Shopper's Bible*, p. 342

layers of the skin and holds it on the surface, which dries the skin from the inside out.

Kaolin
Commonly used in foundations, face powders and dusting powders, kaolin is a fine white clay used in making porcelain. Like bentonite, kaolin smothers and weakens the skin.

Lanolin
A fatty substance extracted from wool, which is frequently found in cosmetics and lotions. Lanolin is a common sensitiser that can cause allergic reactions, such as skin rashes, sometimes due to toxic pesticides present in the sheep's wool. Some sixteen pesticides were identified in lanolin sampled in 1988[124].

Mineral Oil
A derivative of crude oil (petroleum) that is used industrially as a cutting fluid and lubricating oil. Mineral oil forms an oily film over skin to lock in moisture, toxins, and wastes, but hinders normal skin respiration by keeping oxygen out. Used in baby oils.

Petrolatum
A petroleum-based grease that is used industrially as a grease component. Petrolatum exhibits many of the same potentially harmful properties as mineral oil.

Propane
Aerosol propellant. Is flammable and in high doses may be narcotic.

Salt
Very drying, irritating, and corrosive.

Talc
A soft grey-green mineral used in some personal hygiene and cosmetics products. Inhaling talc may be harmful as this substance

---

[124] National Academy of Sciences' concern over lanolin contamination: NRC, 1993, p. 313

is recognised as a potential carcinogen. Talc is widely recognised to be one of the leading causes of ovarian cancer[125].

So what do you do? Where can you go to get hold of safe personal care products that are effective and of high quality?

Samuel Epstein MD, the world-renowned authority on the causes and prevention of cancer, was named the 1998 winner of the Right Livelihood Award (also known as the "Alternative Nobel Prize"). Dr Epstein has devoted the greater part of his life to studying and fighting the causes of cancer. He is Professor of Occupational and Environmental Medicine at the School of Public Health, University of Illinois Medical Center at Chicago, and the chairman of the Cancer Prevention Coalition.

As the author of *The Politics of Cancer* and *The Breast Cancer Prevention Program*, he advocates the use of cosmetics and other products that are free from suspected carcinogens. Based on Dr Epstein's research and recommendations, he has awarded one company the "Seal of Safety" from the Cancer Prevention Coalition. This company, Neways International, manufacturers and distributes its own personal care products, which are free of harmful ingredients. Dr Epstein is enthusiastic about the groundbreaking work Neways has done in this area: *"Neways has pioneered and succeeded in providing consumers with cosmetics and toiletries free of cancer-causing and harmful ingredients and contaminants. I warmly congratulate them on their accomplishments."*

During the course of our work on this book, Credence researchers have had an opportunity to work with Neways technical personnel and examine the Neways product line. I myself have flown to Utah to examine their production plant at Salem and talk with their executives at length. As a result of Credence's investigations, like Dr Epstein, we do not hesitate to recommend Neways' carcinogen-free personal care products and nutritional

---

[125] Steinman, D & Samuel S Epstein *The Safe Shopper's Bible*, p.259

supplements to all who are looking to make a change for the better.

Tom Mower, President of Neways, lays out the focus of his organisation: *"Neways is in the business of helping people detoxify their bodies. Knowing the chemical constituents of your personal care products and their effects on your body enables you to understand how toxic culprits can contaminate your body. Ingredients like sodium lauryl sulfate (SLS), diethanolamine (DEA), triethanolamine (TEA), propylene glycol, fluoride, and alcohol have been identified by experts as known or potential carcinogens that can be found in ordinary personal care products.*

"So Neways provides shampoos without sodium lauryl sulfate. We have lotions without propylene glycol, bubble bath without DEA or TEA, toothpastes without saccharin or fluoride, and mouthwash without alcohol. We use toxin- and carcinogen-free products that give consumers something more than clean skin or fresh breath - they provide peace of mind."

So, let the battle-cry be: Go through the house and toss out all those chemicals. Contact a Neways rep and get those non-toxic substitutes for toothpastes, cosmetics, detergents, polishes, sprays and deodorants, or whole bathroom change-out kits (see *Contacts! Contacts! Contacts!* for further details). Don't use insecticides. Drink bottled water, not tap water. Take a critical look at your lifestyle. Are you puffing away on Marlboros still? Do you drink like Lee Marvin and Oliver Reed at an Oscar celebration? Being sensible about your lifestyle doesn't mean you have to 'Eco Out' and join Greenpeace. Just be smart. Think Hunza.

Now that we have looked at the chemical industry's toxins and how they foist them upon us, it is only fair to answer the sometimes-levelled charge by our establishment mentors that 'wicked' B17 itself is poisonous. What say we to that outrageous assertion?

How Safe is B17?

As previously mentioned, laetrile's arch opponents play heavily on scaring the general public with the institutionalised fear of the word 'cyanide', and yet not a single <u>genuine</u> 'victim' has ever been brought forward to testify to the alleged danger of taking Vitamin B17 naturally. During the past fifty years, many demonstrations have been undertaken to examine the precise mechanisms by which this vitamin acts within the organism to rid it of cancer.

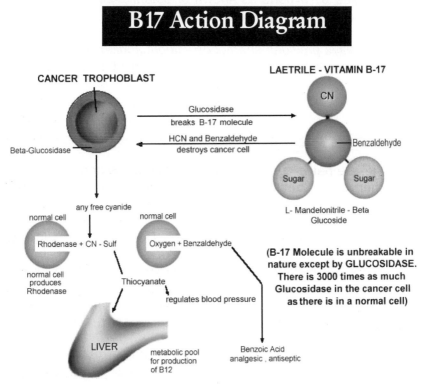

B17 Action Diagram

CANCER TROPHOBLAST

LAETRILE - VITAMIN B-17

CN

Glucosidase
breaks B-17 molecule

HCN and Benzaldehyde
destroys cancer cell

Beta-Glucosidase

Benzaldehyde

Sugar   Sugar

L- Mandelonitrile - Beta
Glucoside

any free cyanide

normal cell   normal cell

Rhodenase + CN - Sulf   Oxygen + Benzaldehyde

normal cell
produces
Rhodenase

Thiocyanate

regulates blood pressure

(B-17 Molecule is unbreakable in
nature except by GLUCOSIDASE.
There is 3000 times as much
Glucosidase in the cancer cell
as there is in a normal cell)

LIVER

metabolic pool
for production
of B12

Benzoic Acid
analgesic , antiseptic

The first thing to note about cyanide is that its compounds are very different from one another. Hydrocyanic acid, which occurs in nature in, for example, the seeds of the common fruits (excluding citrus), is worlds apart from the potassium cyanide used in the gas chamber. The second thing to note is that there is no free hydrogen cyanide floating around in the hydrocyanic acid of the foods we will examine – hydrogen cyanide (HCN) has to be manufactured by the tumour enzyme beta-glucosidase when hydrocyanic acid comes into contact with tumour tissue. Tests show that even when HCN is present in the body in this beneficial reaction, it is harmless to healthy tissue and NON-TOXIC:

Sheep fed the equivalent of 8-10mg of HCN per kilogram per day as linseed meal showed no toxic effects whatsoever[126]. Sheep weighing 66kg were intravenously administered a three-hour dose of 2.7 gms of B17 yielding 300mg of HCN. New Zealand researchers Coop and Blakely reported that *"...at no time during the experiment were even the slightest symptoms observed."* A total of 568mg of HCN was given to a 76kg sheep in the course of an hour. The only symptom the animal showed was *"a general sleepiness for an hour[127]"*. Van der Walt failed to produce chronic poisoning in sheep even after administering 3.2mg HCN/kg daily *for two years[128]*. Worden showed that repeated dosing in rabbits does not produce a cumulative effect and the animal is capable of eliminating excess B17 within two and a half hours.

On the human side, hundreds of thousands each day are now consuming apricot seeds and other B17 derivatives with no problems in defiance of our government stepmothers. This author has been consuming the seeds of apricots, apples, peaches and other fruit for years and has enjoyed paramount health and well-being with no adverse effects whatsoever. Occasionally a nauseous or 'spaced-out' sensation may be experienced by an individual after commencing oral B17 for the first time. This is thought to be the outworkings of the nitriloside effect on corrupted tissue but soon passes. A lower dosage always alleviates such temporary symptoms in cancer sufferers, some of whom have combined B17's selective toxicity to cancer cells with the dynamic

---

[126] **Franklin & Reid** *Australian Veterinary Journal,* 100:92, 1944
[127] **Coop & Blakely** *New Zealand Journal of Science & technology,* 28th February 1949, page 277; ibid, 31:(3)1; ibid, February 1950, page 45)
[128] **Van der Walt** *Veterinary Records,* 52:857, 1940

Metabolic Therapy protocol practised in some of the most successful cancer clinics in the world today[129].

Brown, Wood and Smith observed no toxic effects from consistent B17 usage both in mice and human patients[130]. Maxwell and Bischoff, in studying the possible cumulative effect of HCN in mice, reported, *"After 21 days of exposure to HCN, the red blood cell count and the hemoglobin rose in the mice 12 to 15 percent, and in the rats, 20 to 25 percent[131]."* Interestingly, this experience has been confirmed repeatedly by researchers studying the action of laetrile in advanced cases of human cancer, where reports of pain reduction are frequently heard, due to the analgesic effects of B17's benzaldehyde. Time and time again the evidence shows that B17, when consumed in regulated doses either pharmaceutically (amygdalin/laetrile) as part of the Metabolic Therapy regimen, or as the seed of the apricot or similar, produces anti-neoplastic (anti-cancer) activity in both humans and animals, almost always with no clinical side effects.

Krebs himself tested the safety of B17 in the most dramatic and conclusive manner. In the early 90s, Joe Vialls reported: *"Back in the fifties, Ernst Krebs proved beyond doubt that B17 was completely harmless to humans in the most convincing way possible. After testing the vitamin on animals, he filled a large hypodermic with a mega-dose which he then injected into his own arm. Drastic perhaps, but the adventurous Krebs is still alive and well today[132]."*

Harvey Neufeld, an American B17 nutritionist practising in Mexico, told Credence researchers: *"Most people who are keen to*

---

[129] Metabolic Therapy is a combined regimen of B17, antioxidants, vitamins, minerals and enzymes which boosts the immune system while selectively attacking cancer cells. This treatment, which includes detoxification procedures, has been validated by some of the most successful cancer clinics.

[130] **Brown, Wood & Smith** *Sodium Cyanide as a Cancer Chemotherapeutic Agent... Laboratory and Clinical Studies*, American Journal Obst. & Gynec., 80:907, 1960

[131] **Maxwell & Bischoff** *J Pharmacol. & Exper. Therap., 49:270, 1933*

[132] Vialls, Joe, ibid.

get started with a rich, nitrilosidic diet for prevention purposes want to know how many seeds to take. I would advocate 8-10 apricot or peach seeds a day, eaten along with the fruit, and supplemented with good portions of vegetable greens and general fruit in their diet. I have been doing this for as long as I can remember. Eat an apple, eat the seeds. Eat apricots, crack open the pits and eat out the seeds. Look to get as many nitrilosidic foods into your program as possible[133]. Do the right thing by your body and it will return the favor.

Cancer sufferers would do well to return to a completely natural, detoxifying diet and get as much B17 into their bodies as quickly as possible[134]. Six seeds an hour, or between 40 to 50 seeds a day are adequate to flood the system with B17. Again, lots of fruit and vegetables. 500mg amygdalin tablet supplements are fine too and seem to work well when six a day are taken in conjunction with the 20-30 seeds a day. The idea is to get between 2,000-3,000mg of B17 into the body. In the event that some nausea is experienced, you can back off the dosage a little. Bear in mind though that some nausea is evidence that the hard work is being done.

Some continue with chemo while taking the B17. Chemo works to an extent in tumor reduction, but its toxic effects severely impair the immune system, and we need that to be in good shape to fight on your behalf. I'm not a fan of chemo, but I do recognise that in

---

[133] A highly recommended resource for foods and recipes rich in Vitamin B17 is June de Spain's *The Little Cyanide Cookbook* (available through Credence at www.credence.org). June worked as a toxicologist with the Food & Drug Administration.

[134] An excellent resource for a natural, health detoxifying diet is **Diamond, Harvey & Marilyn** *Fit For Life*, Bantam Books, 1985 – available through Credence Publications at www.credence.org.

certain cases it reduces tumors. But the killing of the cancer? That's down to the selective toxicity of the B17."

Pain, Placebos and Panacea
Examining the Religion of Medicine

Before we close, it is necessary for us to take a brief look at the credibility of today's medical establishment – the same establishment still willing to lie to oppose B17. Credibility always becomes an issue when this vitamin crops up in the conversation, and it really shouldn't. After all, when you get down to the basics of it, the issue of B17 is not one of credibility. All a cancer sufferer wants to know is: *"Does it work or doesn't it? And if it does, will it work for me NOW?"*

Krebs has little time for B17 detractors: *"Scientific truth isn't dependent upon credibility or lack of it. The scientific reality either is or it isn't. And this is the scientific reality - that the seeds of all common fruits (except citrus) contain Vitamin B17, an anti-cancer vitamin."*

Yet since the cancer and general medical establishment are hot to make an issue of credibility, it's only fair in turn to examine their credibility. Let's also talk about the victims of cancer and how they react to their diagnosis. Let's explore too our worship of medicine, for in examining all three together, one can begin putting together a bizarre picture of a public often times desperate to participate in an elaborate religious healing ritual, one in which danger, personal cost to the patient and a potent fear actually appear to be the vital ingredients.

Psychologist and medical researcher Richard Totman studies the effects of faith and suggestion at the heart of our drug-based medical religion today. He has this to say:

"Take anything that is either nasty, expensive or difficult to obtain, wrap it up in mystery and you have a cure."

Have we become the congregation of a medical religion in whose surgery and hospital temples we attempt to seek a kind of redemption? Certainly we take an almost ghoulish delight in telling others what is wrong with us and what our doctors are trying to do to put it right. I remember my daily train journey into London involved enduring the non-stop medical anecdotes of a family friend - what Kevin was suffering from today; what Mary's latest pills were doing for her, and so on. These conversations are an extremely common social interaction, as is apparently the need to endure some kind of sacrifice at the altar of ill-health and emerge bloodied but victorious, thanks to our faith in doctors and their wonderful, life-saving chemical potions.

Do some of us subconsciously make ourselves sick in order to enter this healing/redemption ritual? Judging by the following testimonies from doctors themselves, such a 'blasphemous' notion does not appear to be too wide of the mark.

"I was brought up, as I suppose every physician is, to use placebo[135], bread pills, water injections and other devices... I used to give them by the bushels..."
Professor Richard Cabot, Harvard Medical School, 1903

"Whatever the rights and wrongs, placebo prescribing is widely practised and, if we admit it to ourselves, so is the habit of prescribing for largely social reasons."
Dr K Palmer, British general practitioner, 1998

Not much has changed in 95 years, it seems. Many studies have been conducted examining the effects of placebos. The fact that pharmacologically inert substances such as sugar and bread pills have a measurable clinical effect on illness is proof positive that our healing religion is alive and even kicking into a higher gear today. To illustrate this point, in a television episode of the enthralling series *Trust Me (I'm a Doctor)*, shown on British TV on 11th November 1997, Dr Phil Hammond asked a group to test the strength of a fictional drug he named Ketofenfobraphen. Hammond described the impressive-sounding drug to the group as

---

[135] **placebo** – a harmless, pharmacologically inactive medicine given to a patient which effects 'a cure'.

'a powerful new painkiller that works by selectively blocking the effects of prostaglandin 2 alpha'.

"It's been licensed in the USA and Japan for a year," Hammond enthusiastically told his volunteers, *"and sales have gone through the roof. In fact, I'd recommend you to buy shares in the company. Its beauty is that it works quickly – usually within ten minutes – although it can occasionally give you a dry mouth and make you feel dizzy. Mind you, it's expensive – seven tablets for £14.99 and they do not taste very nice – but it's the best drug in its class and I use it all the time for my knee. And when the British Lions were on tour in South Africa, they insisted on having some flown out especially..."* etc. etc.

Note that in giving out the details of Ketofenfobraphen, Dr Hammond is careful to mention each aspect which will affect the outcome of the healing ritual: The drug is a 'wonder drug'. It is officially sanctioned (licensed). It produces side effects (dry mouth and dizziness). It is horribly expensive and has an unpleasant taste. And lastly, a group most of us look up to (the British Lions) think it's the business.

The volunteers were randomly split into two groups after being told they would receive either Ketofenfobraphen or a placebo. In reality both groups were given different coloured placebos. Ten minutes after taking the tablets, they were blindfolded and asked to submerge a hand in ice and pull it out only when it got uncomfortably painful. Hammond reports that after five minutes, twice as many volunteers who thought they had been given the painkiller still had their hands in ice:

"When I asked if anyone had suffered side effects as a result of taking the 'powerful painkillers', one woman said she had felt faint and dizzy soon after swallowing the pills[136]."

We hear cries of 'quackery!' levelled by the medical establishment against treatments unsanctioned by them and yet

---

[136] **Hammond, Dr Phil** *Trust Me (I'm a Doctor)*, Metro Books, 1999 p.91 ISBN 1900512602

official quackery on a vast scale, in some cases involving highly toxic and deadly drugs, surrounds us in breathtaking abundance. Got a pain? Have a drug. Got a headache? Have a drug. Got a bad attitude? Have a drug. When the only tool you have is a hammer, very soon everything starts looking like a nail. The pharmaceutical industry cynically ignores unprofitable prevention in favour of successfully snowing us that biotechnology is the future for mankind's health. I beg to differ. I think, if we are not prudent and quick, biotechnology will be the ruin of us. It already contributes to the leading cause of death in the Western world, as we found out earlier.

Also, as we are discovering, and as Ralph Nader and many others have found out, 'orthodox' medical quackery has created sickness and death on a scale that is hard for us to accept at first, but the true picture is beginning to emerge along with the scandals and hard statistics which show us where the real problem lies.

Have we become like the shade-tree mechanic who spends so much time tinkering with his car that it no longer runs the way it used to? Professor Chris Bulstrode, an orthopaedic surgeon turned medical teacher, puts the compelling case for *less* doctors and medicine, not more:

"More doctors just means more illness. If we want a healthier and happier country, we should get rid of a lot of doctors. I cannot have been the only person who was absolutely incensed to discover that when the Berlin Wall came down, the military strength of the Eastern Block was an order of magnitude less than we had been led to believe. I want to try all the Western generals for lying to the public about how strong the Russians were. These generals have done three things over the last thirty years. They have frightened the hell out of the Russians, they have frightened the hell out of us, and they have stolen a huge amount of money from the budget that could have been used elsewhere. As I was thinking about this, I realized that this is exactly what we as doctors do in health care."

So how does this medical and drug tinkering apply to cancer? A person receiving a cancer diagnosis for the first time is a frightened individual. Cancer has been bred into us as the secret fear at the back of the 20th century mind, the Sword of Damocles come to destroy our family, corrupting our vitals a little each day, to rob a little boy of his mother, a daughter of her father. Yet cancer also remains a potent social stigma, despite its abundance, causing relatives and friends politely to distance themselves in some cases from the unfortunate sufferer in question.

Who doesn't hate the idea of a hospital? Who doesn't fear the fateful diagnosis of the oncologist? Cancer victims are pitied as much today as they ever were in decades past because cancer still seems insurmountable and frightening (*"Jack's got cancer." "Oh, well. That's it for him then."*). More often than not, cancer victims sense an isolation; realise that something has changed that won't ever be the same again. They know almost nothing about the circumstances surrounding the cause or onset of their illness, and so they turn to the easy familiarity of their local doctor or mainstream medical consultant who they hope will offer some comfort and a way out.

Thus the cancer victim enters the medical ritual. The procedure that follows runs a well-worn and predictable path in orthodox medicine. The instillation of fear. The patient enters a foreign environment of strange words, stranger machines and the strangest smells. A biopsy or similar operation to test for tumour malignancy followed by the commencement of surgery, chemo- or radiotherapy. Sometimes the life of the patient is extended or shortened by some months. Sometimes surgery cuts out the tumour without spreading the cancer. Sometimes it doesn't. More often than not the resultant chemotherapy or radiation treatment poisons or burns the patient's immune system, liver and kidneys into complete submission before the cancer itself closes for the kill.[137]

---

[137] Many doctors practising Metabolic Therapy have told Credence researchers that almost all patients who come to them with cancer in its advanced stages have impaired liver function due to the treatments that have been given to them in the name of 'advanced cancer science'. Thus these doctors have become adept

Cancer patients who do stride out on their own to investigate the alternatives to orthodox treatments become bewildered and disheartened by the rainbow of cure-alls and snake-oil remedies confronting them. Yes, even in the realm of alternative health there are the true quacks. All promise long life and happiness and some cost a small fortune. Often times, the intrepid patient will discuss alternative therapies with their doctor who understands their emotional need to search, but who tactfully reminds them of all the work being done by the pharmaceutical companies to cure their condition.

No one would seriously blame doctors for the woes of the world, or even for their failure to cure cancer in our loved ones. These busy and overworked ones have barely enough hours in the day to do what they have to do. And this is, in itself, the tragedy of where we have arrived as a society. In a commercial environment where the life and health stakes are high and doctors have to rely on medical briefing packages prepared for them, what becomes of the rest of us when part of the industry-accepted science in which they were trained is so tragically flawed?

Some reading this book will have their hopes raised by the information contained within it, only to have them dashed when they excitedly broach the B17/Metabolic Therapy subject with their doctors, the majority of whom we must remember were trained, rightly or wrongly, in allopathic medical institutions funded by the pharmaceutical companies. The 'establishment' responses from GPs and oncologists usually go something like this:

"Ah, laetrile! That old wife's tale! Doesn't work. Never has done. We disproved that one back in the '70s, Mr Smith. It's cyanide, for goodness sake!"

---

at using nutritional procedures to recover liver function prior to treating their patients' cancers with the protocol.

Or: "If B17 really worked, Mrs Winterbottom, don't you think we'd be prescribing it and the good news would be all over the newspapers?"

But nutritional therapy for cancer can never be part of the orthodox healing ritual for four reasons. It cannot be patented. The mystery of cancer and its treatment would evaporate. The drug establishment and cancer charities would be cut out of the profit loop and our grocers would become our new doctors! An end would come to the fear which binds the followers to the medical religion.

Not all doctors, as we have seen, are negative to nutritional therapy. Some, as we shall see in a minute, have become curious and excited in cases where their patient's 'miracle' regression can be provably put down to nutritional therapy - in other words, after the patient has ceased all conventional treatment to return home to die or, as the cancer establishment puts it, 'to enjoy a remaining quality of life'.

Nearly all GPs have an honest heart and are desperately involved with their patient's struggle for survival (the heroes of the B17 story are almost all doctors). As we have seen from the oncologists and biochemists quoted earlier, more than a few have noticed with despair the inability of orthodox treatments to arrest cancer and so are willing to take a fresh look at the alternatives. Those who have taken the trouble to do their homework recognise that Krebs' and Sugiura's research on B17 *is* based on solid science and there is nothing sensible to gainsay it. As a result, official medical attitudes towards cancer are changing, but tragically not fast enough to save a lot of us at the present time.

The point that needs to be made and fully understood here is this. Hard though it may be for most of us to accept, doctors and the medical establishment are as fallibly human as the rest of us. PhDs don't stop greed, nor do the letters 'MD' guarantee a perfect and impartial diagnosis. This hasn't stopped an institutionalised medical arrogance automatically rearing its offended head when non-sanctioned treatments that work with cancer challenge accepted dogma. Can doctors and the medical establishment *always* be trusted to know what's right for us? Not in all cases. Richard Smith put it this way in March 1997:

"Doctors are set apart. We are a priesthood with our own rites, beliefs, systems of initiation and tribal practices. And we have special powers. The public turns to us in moments of extremity and expects an answer, even a solution. Often we cannot provide it..."

And that from the editor of the *British Medical Journal*!

Traditional medicine is increasingly coming under fire as cracks appear in the flawless picture we have painted of our medicinal saviours. When *Trust Me (I'm a Doctor)* – the book and the TV series written by Dr Phil Hammond and Michael Mosley - came before the British public, the British National Health Service (NHS) and private medical practice were portrayed in a strange new, disturbingly dark and foreboding light. Dr Hammond remarks:

"In BBC2's 'Cardiac Arrest', an NHS hospital was depicted as a war zone, with staff bullying one another, humiliating patients and taking the path of least resistance in order to survive. The only way to cope was not to care. For the first time in a British TV program, nurses were portrayed as a bunch of clock-watching, bolshy witches, and the rougher side of doctors was shown... one making easily overhead remarks about a man with lung cancer ("He's got so much asbestos in him, it'll take a year to cremate him.") A bullied female doctor with an alcohol problem committed suicide. All very bleak and unsettling[138,139]."

The picture painted by most who have worked in the National Health Service is one in which overworked and inexperienced junior doctors are engaged in a daily struggle to keep their heads

---

[138] Hammond, Dr Phil *Trust Me (I'm a Doctor)*, ibid.

[139] *Cardiac Arrest* was generally popular among doctors. One survey showed that junior doctors believed the program was an accurate portrayal of their working conditions (*BMJ*, 1994, vol. 309, p.132).

above crushing workloads. Some of these believe their problems started during medical school, where they were first introduced to the deeply ingrained cronyism and party culture of the medical establishment.

Two surveys, reported in *The Lancet*, discovered that heavy drinking and illicit drug use were common among second-year medical students, and that these invariably increased after graduation[140]. Of the 90 house officers studied, 60% of both sexes exceeded their safe limits. 35% of men and 10% of women reported using other drugs such as hallucinogenic mushrooms, LSD, ecstasy, amyl nitrite, cocaine and amphetamines. As for their mental state, 21 percent of men and 45 percent of women had anxiety scores indicating possible pathological anxiety.

Stress too was to be a major factor in influencing the later mental conditions and competence of doctors when interacting with their patients. In 1991, a study of doctors who qualified in 1986 found that 58% of men and 76% of women regretted entering medicine[141].

Dr Hammond states: *"Drinking and drug abuse are clearly coping mechanisms picked up in medical school, but it is impossible to predict which of the many heavy student drinkers will go on to develop a problem. The BMA estimated that up to 13,000 practising UK doctors are addicted to drugs or alcohol. If each makes 2,000 clinical decisions a year, at a conservative estimate, that is 26 million decisions affecting patient care* [including prescribing potentially lethal drugs] *made by doctors who can't function without alcohol or other drugs[142]."*

Doctors often neglect to advise their patients of their true condition. Patients are usually frightened and in awe and tend not to ask for an interpreter when their consultants revert to medical jargon, with predictable and unfortunate consequences. A study of

[140] *Lancet*, 1996, vol. 348, pp.922-925; 1998, vol. 352, p.785
[141] **Allen, Isobel** *Doctors and their Careers: A New Generation*, London: Policies Studies Institute, 1988
[142] Hammond, Dr Phil, ibid.

100 patients interviewed within five days of major abdominal surgery found that 27 didn't know which organ had been removed and 44 were unaware of the exact nature of the surgical procedure, despite having been counselled before the operation[143].

Neither do doctors appear to be as in control of emergency events as *Casualty* and *ER* would have the public believe. A Cardiff Royal Infirmary study polled 113 doctors in cardiac arrest teams from 62 teaching and district general hospitals in England and Wales. Only 32 could cite the full sequence of managing ventricular fibrillation (the commonest cause of cardiac arrest) and 32 didn't even know the initial actions to take[144].

The medical establishment bravely dons the mask of unflappable capability, and yet the statistics imply a worldwide allopathic disaster is occurring. *Trust Me* reports that between 4-13% of admissions to hospital in the United States are due to medical accidents. 7% of these patients suffer permanent damage and 14% die. In England, where there are about 8 million admissions a year, even the lower figure extrapolates to 320,000 medical accidents a year, resulting in 40,000 deaths and 20,000 cases of permanent disability.

And orthodox medicine is the one crying 'quackery'?

Dispelling the myth we have been sold that doctors are society's guardian angels and above medical reproach, scandals abound within the NHS of chronic bed shortages, patients being treated on trolleys in corridors and bungled medical procedures occurring far more frequently than the public realises. Surgeons occasionally pick up names like 'Chopper', 'Slasher' or 'Hacker'. Rodney Ledward, a Kent gynaecologist, was struck off by the General Medical Council in September 1998. Known as 'The Butcher' by his colleagues, he nevertheless was able to practise his incompetence *for sixteen years* before he was eventually

---

[143] *British Medical Journal*, 1988, vol. 296, pp. 839-840
[144] *British Medical Journal*, vol. 309, pp. 1408-1409

stopped. Most of his colleagues knew of his ineptitude but were unwilling to be the ones to blow the whistle. As a result of their silence, hundreds of women today bear the scars from the hacking of a doctor who once boasted he was 'the fastest gynaecologist in the South East', having on one occasion completed seven hysterectomies between 8am and noon.

On 23rd March 1999, the front-page news in England told the tale of Anita Froggart who had a breast removed after being wrongly diagnosed as a cancer victim. Doctors later admitted that a sample of her healthy tissue had been mixed up with one from a cancer patient.

At the time of writing, the Bristol Royal Infirmary is the target of a £15 million General Medical Council enquiry that will rock the foundations of British medical practice for years to come. Several hundred babies are believed to have perished or were maimed after botched cardiac procedures by incompetent surgeons, producing such an inordinately high mortality rate that the institution was referred to among consultants for years as 'The Killing Fields' or 'The Departure Lounge'. Even though GPs would go out of their way to refer their patients away from Bristol to other areas, once again nothing official was done. Whistle-blowing Bristol nurse Helen Stratton later reported:

"Parents used to say, "See you later!" to their children and I used to stand there thinking, "No, you won't.[145]*"*

So is our medical establishment above reproach? Hardly. *But the irony is, most doctors know it even if the public doesn't.* Yes, doctors are necessary and a valuable part of our society. But what are we to make of the scandals which rob us of our loved ones when so much can be done to stop these senseless tragedies from happening? As Ernst Krebs remarks, you're a pretty rotten expert if you die from the very diseases you are trying to prevent in others. Sad though it may be to accept, we do have cardiologists dying of

---

[145] *Health Service Journal,* 4th June 1998

heart attacks, neurosurgeons succumbing to strokes, osteologists dying of osteoporosis and, yes, oncologists perishing from cancer.

I believe though that the real tragedy of cancer lies not just with our overworked doctors and their deeply flawed establishment, but with us. Most ordinary citizens gave up looking after themselves years ago and moved the responsibility to BUPA, Blue Shield and the government to do it for them. Now society's general perception is that our doctors constitute our first and last line of defence against any crippling illness and we cannot survive without them. This is baloney. Once upon a time, no one had medical insurance. Hard to believe, but there you go.

Of course, true and responsible medicine has a part to play in our society today - no question of it. Every time I fell off my motorcycle as a teenager, I was grateful to the Accident & Emergency Unit for stitching me back together again with great skill, a kind word and some marvellous coffee. Certain ailments are best treated in our hospitals – who would argue? But when is enough enough? Is it when medicine ceases to be for the good of the patient and begins operating for the good of the shareholder? If it is, we are way past that point today, and our health industries have become ever more cynical and manipulative in their dealings with their patients' misery and weakness as time progresses.

As for our worship of drugs and all things medical, I beg to remind you that the great George Washington was bled to death in 1797 by some of the most well-educated medical practitioners of his day. No doubt, had you been at the august president's deathbed raising a fuss as they slashed his wrists, these learned professionals would have angrily turned on you: *"We know what we're doing. We're DOCTORS!"* The men who killed George Washington were extremely intelligent. They were experienced practitioners who were no doubt highly educated. They were also wrong.

If cancer seems mysterious and frightening, that is because society has packaged it that way. But the reality is, humankind has been ravaged in the past by those supposedly insurmountable environmental diseases we looked at earlier, and these have been beaten by nothing more controversial than a change in diet, a change in environment and a simple vitamin. To our ancestors living back then, these diseases seemed every bit as complicated and terrifying as cancer appears to us today. But the names of these diseases are all but out of the modern dictionary. So why not cancer?

METABOLIC DISEASES

Disease	Prevented by	Death Rate[146]	Status
Scurvy	Vitamin C (ascorbic)	varies	Defeated
Pellagra	Vitamin B3 (niacin)	97%	Defeated
P. Anemia	Vitamin B12 (& folic acid)	99%	Defeated
Beriberi	Vitamin B1 (thiamine)	-	Defeated
Cancer	**Vitamin B17 (laetrile)**	**varies**	Defeated

When man rids himself of the delusion that a complicated-looking and horrendous disease requires an equally complicated, horrendous (and expensive) treatment in order to cure it, we can then return to sanity. And what is sanity? Is sanity not gauged by the reaction of the man facing an overflowing sink? Will he reach for the mop or the tap?

Today, because of the religion of medicine, billions are spent on *cure* and a minuscule amount by comparison on *prevention*, and so we are constantly mopping. Our diets are vitamin- and mineral-deficient, and even as we scoff all that haûte cuisine in the world's finest restaurants, convincing ourselves we are so civilised, we are living the real insanity in a world we are increasingly polluting with every new step of our technology. Our bodies cannot appreciate the decor of a five-star restaurant, they only react to what comes down the gullet in the form of nutrition. Most of us are still running the gasoline car on diesel. We are, quite literally, what we eat.

---

[146] Expected mortality rate at the time, once diagnosed.

Imagine if the government told us that, in order to improve road safety statistics, it was going to remove seatbelts from cars, ban airbags, outlaw anti-lock brakes, repeal the baby-seat laws and instead pour millions into teaching doctors how to fix the resultant broken heads in the hospitals. If this were to happen, Members of Parliament or Congressmen would be dragged outside by an outraged public and given the good news in the parking lot in no uncertain terms, and yet this attitude is the unbelievable state of affairs in healthcare today.

Of course we see the token gestures made by our leaders towards educating us in disease prevention. I worked in advertising, I used to see their pathetic campaigns (*"Eat those fruits and vegetables, kids!"*). The sorry truth is, the prevention ethic doesn't bring in tax revenues from drug licensing, nor does it find a way of replacing the incredible incomes governments receive taxing tobacco and alcohol. Ironically We the People know cigarettes and whisky are bad for us, and so in our guilt and naughtiness we don't mind forking out the government tax on them. Look me in the eye and tell me we're not certifiable already with this kind of attitude.

The most deadly items to our health are those we put into our supermarket carts. Stop and think next time you go shopping. Many products masquerading as personal and household care items contain chemical toxins that are known carcinogens. Much of the food now available is nothing more than highly processed commercial material passed off to the public as edible matter. And here am I, from the bottom of my heart, telling you, "Don't trust others to look out for your health! Do it yourself!" The latest farce with the introduction of genetically modified foods should convince you of ulterior corporate agendas even if the foregoing chapters haven't. We must become good at prevention *ourselves* and look after our families. It takes only a little common sense and a small degree of consistency. If we simply turn off the tap, we will avoid the flood.

Researcher and author Paul B Rogerson comments: *"In my experience, the great majority of those who learn about B17 say, "Wow, that's neat!" and then proceed to do nothing to change their dietary regimen. And so inevitably these folks will form part of the cancer statistics of the future. What a sad indictment on our civilisation that we have become too fond of our gluttonous habits, too lazy in our self-discipline, too apathetic with our leaders and their agendas, that even when faced with such monumentally good news as this, in the final analysis most of us are not going to do anything to save ourselves.*[147]*."*

In his book, *World Without Cancer,* Edward Griffin summarises his findings on four available treatments for cancer:

SURGERY: Least harmful. Sometimes a life-saving, stop-gap measure. No evidence that patients who receive radical or extensive surgical options live any longer than those who receive the most conservative options, or, for that matter, those who receive none at all. Believed to increase the likelihood of disseminating cancer to other locations.

When dealing with internal tumors affecting reproductive or vital organs, the statistical rate of long-term survival is, on the average, 10—15%. After metastasis, the statistical chances for long-term survival are close to zero.

RADIOLOGY: The burning out of tumors using x-rays. Very harmful in many ways. Spreads the cancer and weakens the patient's resistance to other diseases. Serious and painful side-effects, including heart failure. No evidence that treated patients live any longer, on the average, than those not treated. Statistical rate of long-term survival after metastasis is close to zero.

CHEMOTHERAPY: Toxic drug therapy. Also spreads the cancer through weakening of immunological defense mechanism plus general toxicity. Leaves patient susceptible to other diseases and infections, often leading to death from these causes.

---

[147] **Rogerson, Paul** *The Final Assault on the Big C*, a written commentary, The Ludlow Reader, Ventura, California USA

Extremely serious side-effects. No evidence that treated patients live any longer, on the average, than untreated patients. Statistical rate of long-term survival after metastasis is close to zero.

VITAMIN [METABOLIC] THERAPY: B17 seeds, laetrile/amygdalin tablets or laetrile administered intravenously. Non-toxic. Side effects include increased appetite, weight gain, and lowered blood pressure. Eliminates or sharply reduces pain without narcotics. Is a natural substance found in foods and is compatible with human biological experience. Destroys cancer cells while nourishing non-cancer cells[148].

[148] Griffin, G Edward, ibid.

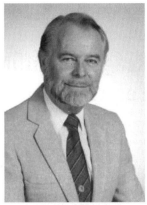

G Edward Griffin
Author of *World Without Cancer*

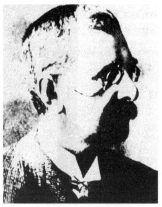

Prof. John Beard
Wrote the Trophoblastic Thesis of Cancer proposing that cancer was a healing process that simply wasn't terminating upon completion of the task

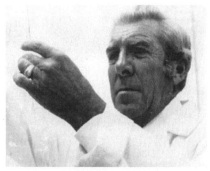

Dr Harold Manner
One of the key medical figures who formulated nutritional therapy for cancer

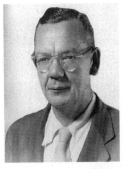

Dr Ian MacDonald
The prominent cancer surgeon quoted in *Who's Who*, who was co-author of the establishment's California Report, which stated that laetrile was useless in the treatment of cancer

Dr Henry Garland
Co-author with MacDonald of the California Report

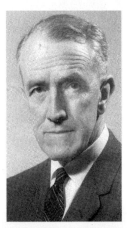

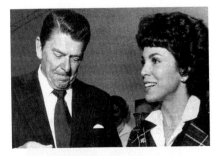

Reagan Reaffirms Laetrile Backing

Even as federal bureaucrats were trying to bury Laetrile with a rigged report, President Reagan was reasserting his view that people should be free to use the substance.

EXCLUSIVE TO SPOTLIGHT
By Mike Blair

President Reagan was one of many politicians who asserted the people's right to laetrile as a cancer treatment, if that was their wish. Many cancer establishment insiders had grave reservations about the way in which laetrile was being summarily dismissed

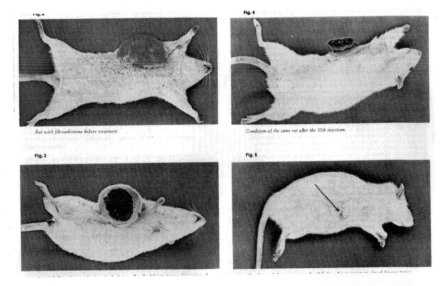

Fig. 4

Rat with fibroadenoma before treatment.

Condition of the same rat after the 10th injection.

Fig. 3

Fig. 5

ENZYME THERAPY ('knifeless surgery') - In the 1970s, the WOBE-MUGOS enzyme tests repeatedly and dramatically demonstrated the effect of proteolytic enzymes on a rat's fibroadenoma during a 40-day period. In Metabolic Therapy, this enzyme action is coupled with emulsified Vitamin A, B17/amygdalin and detoxification procedures aggressively to assault a human patient's malignant cells.

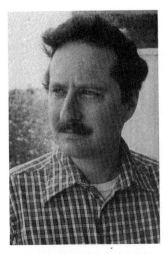

Dr Ralph Moss, erstwhile member of the Sloan-Kettering team, spoke out about the mis-reporting of Dr Sugiura's laetrile trials. Dr Moss was later fired from his position when he convened a press conference to release the true details of Dr Sugiura's findings

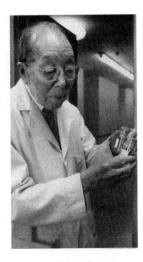

Dr Kanematsu Sugiura
Arguably America's most experienced cancer researcher in the 1970s, conducted a five-year series of trials on B17 at Memorial Sloan Kettering in New York. To the outrage of his peers, he reported that amygdalin B17 in his opinion was the most effective anti-cancer agent he had tested

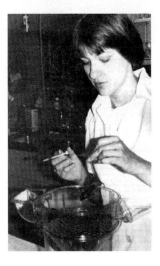

Maria Manhardt
A Loyola graduate and the Manner team's 'mousekeeper', prepares to give one of the subjects its amygdalin injection. Mice treated with the B17/enzyme/vitamin cocktail always demonstrated a noticeably finer physical condition than the control group. Rats with brain tumours would later show marked improvements with treatments of a B17-rich cassava treatment, carried out by Professor Monica Hughes of Newcastle University, UK

A lab victory over breast cancer

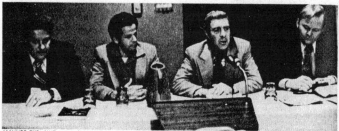

MANNER EXPLAINS — Loyola biologist Harold Manner, Ph.D., told the press in Newark, N.J., how he and a Loyola team of graduate students achieved a 100% response with the metabolic treatment of breast cancer in mice. With him at the Committee-sponsored doctors' workshop were, from left, Harold Harper, M.D., CHOICE Editor Mike Culbert, and Committee President Robert W. Bradford.

—PAT MURPHY PHOTO

Scientific Support from
Loyola For Krebs' Laetrile

Dr HW Manner announces his breakthrough in cancer research at the National Health Federation Press conference held in Chicago in September 1977. *"Laetrile alone won't do it,"* said Manner. *"But enzyme/vitamin/laetrile therapy destroys cancer."* Metabolic Therapy is born.

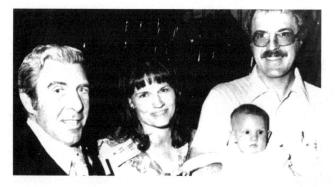

Dr Manner introducing Ann and Jim Metcalfe at the 6th Annual Cancer Convention. Ann, who is a cancer patient, continued to take Metabolic Therapy treatments throughout her pregnancy. Her baby was born in a healthier condition than any of their other children.

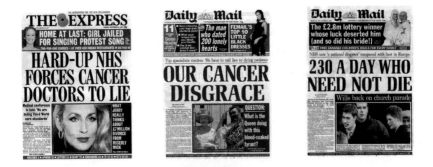

The more things change, the more they stay the same:
Even today, orthodox medicine is ridden with cancer scandals,
treatments and screening procedures that are proven failures.
On the other hand, sensible cancer prevention procedures and
nutritional cancer treatment alternatives such as B17 Metabolic
Therapy, which have enjoyed decades of success in foreign
clinics, are either scorned outright or cynically ignored.

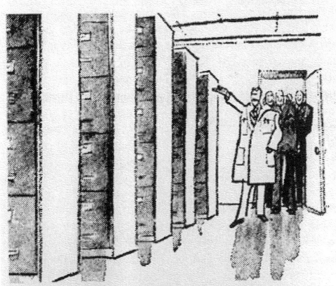

*"There's where we keep all the unpublished reports on
Laetrile"*

—FROM A CARTOON IN *SECOND OPINION*

Vitamin A Can Prevent and Cure Cancer—But 1 American In 3 Doesn't Get Enough of It

Proteolytic Enzymes and Megadoses of Vitamin A in Cancer Therapy

M. Wolf, K. Maehder, E. v. Pirozzi, K. Rausberger, O. Weigelt und F. We

Presented before: The Mexican Cancer Congress, Sept. 30, 1971, Mexico

ong other biochemical compounds, vitamin A has become very important

investigations of different research centers

and mou...
"Recent dru.......
have opened up a who..
"With vitamin A therapy, w..

...ment with vitamin A reverses the
leading American universi-

...ngly, nearly
...f vitamin A
...le to cancer-

...nal needs. It is

VITAMIN A
ARROTS CUT LUNG CANCER

n Feb. 7, 1981, *United Press*
national reported that the
ident of the *British Associa-*
for Cancer Research said a
heavy with carrots may help
ice the risk of contracting
cancer by as much as 40 per

. Richard Doll said his latest re-
h shows there is a definite link be-
t reduced cancer risk and the form
amin A found in carrots, carotene.
believe there is now a light at the

blood level. Then over a period of years,
scientists would study their cancer incidence compared to a group that received no supplementary vitamin A.

In a refreshing departure from past
rhetoric, NCI's Breslow said:

"Until now we have been approaching
cancer from the st---dpoint of destroy-
ing it by surgery,
therapy. The exc
have evidence we
physiologically t
processes."

Carrot juice, in
it l

KREBS EXPLAINS VIT. B-17, SEES BRIGHTER FUTURE

...o — In 1952 Dr. Ern
... and leadir

Biologist says Cancer Can Be Cured, Avoided by Diet

By Kathy Titchen
Star-Bulletin Writer

Sarah Sockett and Dr. Ernesto Contreras, Sr.

"I've been free of cancer since 1991.
I love God and I love my doctor!"

Sarah

Biologist Waging Fight To Vindicate Laetrile

Claim 'Major Breakthrough' in Treatment of Cancer With Enzymes and Vitamin A

By DONALD HUDSON

Two West German physicians
have claimed a "major breakthrough" in treating several ma-

cancers have completely disappeared,
he said.

"We have found also that enzyme-
vitamin A therapy achieves improved

OK, SO WHAT CAN I DO NOW?

Here we are at the halfway mark! Up to now, we have been looking at cancer and the background to the phenomenon of nutritional therapy for cancer – its medical and political history. Now we are going to look at nutritional therapy and prevention in more detail, how the whole program works, and what each individual component brings to the battle against cancer and ill-health.

Generally three types of people read this book and each has a different path he or she might wish to consider taking:

I WANT TO LEARN ABOUT PREVENTION

If you do not have cancer, but want to learn about cancer prevention and how the Neways program and nutritional therapy prevention can give you and your family an exceptionally high degree of protection, not just from cancer, but from a whole range of serious illnesses, there is a section especially for you coming up a little later on.

I WANT TO LEARN ABOUT NUTRITIONAL THERAPY

If you have been diagnosed with cancer and want to find out what the clinics and even those at home have been doing with nutritional therapy, all the detailed information you will need is coming up in the next sections. Please let me stress at this point as I did at the beginning that cancer is of course a serious condition and a qualified health practitioner should always be consulted in the matter of which treatments you decide to take. For this reason, I am also going to point you in the direction of qualified medical personnel who have been practising nutritional therapy for cancer for many years with great results, who are on hand to answer any remaining questions you may have at the conclusion of this book.

I WANT TO DO MORE RESEARCH

If you want to learn more details on nutritional treatments for cancer than we have been able to provide in this book, a bibliography and extended reading and contact list are provided in the final pages.

125

The next sections are in appendix format and are recommended for each of the above reader groups. Please study them carefully. Firstly, we hear from Dr Krebs himself regarding the broader points of his research and his comments on various topics. Next, the Frequently Asked Questions (FAQs) section nails some of the common queries about nutritional therapy. After that, a section is devoted to the most popular and, in my personal view, effective strategy for fighting cancer – B17 Metabolic Therapy.

Then we hear from Tina Cooke and Hilary Englefield, who reversed their breast cancer by undergoing Metabolic Therapy. Both now head up UK organisations devoted to broadcasting the great news on the alternative, non-allopathic approaches to cancer treatment.

Lastly, a report from the trenches with Health Genesis Inc's David Arjona, Christian Brothers' Jason Vale and myself, who have daily contact with those who are going the B17 route with their treatment. Jason is himself a prior cancer sufferer who ridded himself of the condition with peach seeds! Since recovering, he has appeared on NBC, in various newspapers and today hosts an Internet journal reporting the amazing testimonies of those who took the B17 information and ran with it. These stories will be an inspiration to you.

Finally, I have enclosed a contact fact sheet on addresses, web-sites and telephone numbers that readers will want to keep handy for more information on this fascinating subject. I receive e-mails and letters all the time from readers who want to share their stories with others. I would love to hear from you too!

I predict that the storm against nutritional treatments for cancer, and in particular our little friend B17, will continue as before, of course. Watch out for the fly-on-the-wall TV documentaries pillorying B17, apricot seeds and exposing the 'sad' and gullible people who believe all this 'vitamin quackery!' Please make up your own mind based on the evidence. Sooner or later, we must all rediscover our common sense and start looking after ourselves. My earnest hope for all who have taken the trouble to read this book and ponder its contents is that you will, like many others now across the world, set your hand to the task, along with your doctors, and help bury this scourge of cancer forever.

OK. Without further ado, let's proceed....

Ernst Krebs Speaks

Taken from a 1974 speech presented before the Second Annual Cancer Convention at the Ambassador Hotel in Los Angeles, California.

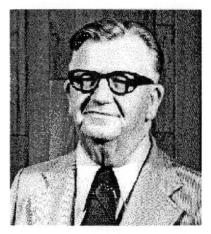

"It is certainly a pleasure to be here at the Second Annual Convention of the Cancer Control Society - an outgrowth, as you know, of the International Association of Cancer Victims and Friends.

As I look back through the years marking the emergence of these two fine societies, I can recall the number of miraculous victories we have had in those intervening years; that it is as true today as it was eleven years ago that laetrile, Vitamin B17, is the first and last final hope in the prophylacsis in therapy of cancer in man and animals. The reason for this is that laetrile is a vitamin. It is the 17th of the B vitamins.

We hear a great deal about its use in terminal cancer, but the time to start with Vitamin B17 is now before the disease becomes clinical. The time to start is the same with any matter of adequate nutrition and that is right now. You may start now by commencing to eat the seeds of all common fruits that you eat. Apricot and peach seeds contain almost 2 percent of Vitamin B17 by weight. The apple seed, although very small, is equally rich in Vitamin B17 - so are the seeds of prunes, plums, cherries, and nectarines. The only common fruits on the hemisphere that lack nitrilosidic seeds are the citrus fruits. This lack has come about by artificial cultivation, by breeding and hybridization, since the seeds of citrus fruits on the African continent still contain Vitamin B17.

Two more rich sources of Vitamin B17 are the simple cereal millet and buckwheat. Macadamia nuts, although expensive and exotic, are very rich in Vitamin B17 and so are bamboo shoots, mung beans, lima beans, butter beans and certain strains of garden peas. But for convenience, the simple source for your Vitamin B17 are the seeds of the common fruit.

We know something about the prophylactic dose of Vitamin B17. For example, we know the Hunzas represent a population that has been cancer-free for over 900 years of its existence. This population has a natural diet which supplies on the average between 50 to 75 milligrams of Vitamin B17 a day.

Hunzaland is a land that has sometimes been described as the 'place where the apricot is king.' The Hunzakuts eat the fresh apricots for the three months they are in season and the remainder of the year they eat dried apricots. They never eat a dried apricot without enclosing the seed. This supplies them with better than the average of 50 to 75 milligrams of Vitamin B17 a day.

There are many of us in the western world who don't ingest this amount of Vitamin B17 in the course of an entire year. As a result we're in the midst of a fulminating deficiency of Vitamin B17 or nitriloside, the anti-neoplastic vitamin. Its absence from our diets accounts for the fact that cancer within our population has reached such a pandemisity as to account for its occurrence in one in every three American families. The occurrence is probably much greater than that because it is very late in its development when the cancer is detected. Many who develop cancer are killed by accident or intercurrent diseases before the malignant process has become sufficiently advanced to cause them to have it diagnosed.

Cancer is a chronic, metabolic disease - that is obvious. It isn't an infectious disease, which is caused by bacteria or viruses. It is a disease that is metabolic in origin. A metabolic disease is a disease that is wedded to our utilization of food. Most metabolic diseases have as their basis the deficiency of specific vitamins and minerals.

Let me give you a categorical or axiomatic truth to take with you - one that is totally uncontradictable, scientifically, historically and in every other way. This is, that no chronic or metabolic disease in the history of medicines has ever been prevented or cured except by factors normal to the diet or normal to the animal economy. There have been many erstwhile fatal and devastating diseases that now have become virtually unknown. They have been prevented and cured by ingesting the dietary factors and thereby preventing the deficiencies which accounted for these diseases.

The one with which you are probably most familiar is scurvy - a fatal disease that killed mankind by the thousands; a disease that would sometimes wipe out an entire polar expedition. Scurvy accounted for about 50 percent mortality among the Crusaders. It is a disease that can be totally prevented and cured with Vitamin C or ascorbic acid - a factor normal to an adequate diet. As you know so well from your school days, Great Britain acquired the dominion of the seas by discovering that through adding lime or other citrus juices to the provisions of the British mariners, the curse of scurvy from the British sea power was removed. Therefore Britain competitively gained the ascendancy on the seas. Prior to the incorporation of Vitamin C into their diets, it wasn't uncommon for three-fourths of the crew to become seriously ill by the end of a voyage and then those who didn't die would mysteriously recover after hitting shore because they would have access to fresh fruits and vegetables rich in Vitamin C.

Then we have pernicious anemia, which had a mortality rate of 98 or 99 percent and no medical modality under the sun could touch it. Arsenic and its salts, strychnine, iron and hundreds of other remedies were tried but to no avail until the researchers Drs. Murphy, Shipple and Minot commenced their classical studies on the relationship of pernicious anemia to dietary deficiency.

While working at the University of California they discovered a very simple remedy for preventing and curing this disease. They simply said to their patients, "Go down to your butcher shop and get a quarter pound of fresh liver. Grind it up and take a tablespoon everyday and take the quarter pound and cook it very lightly and just singe the surface and use this as a ration for three days." And when the patients followed this advice without exception, those with pernicious anemia made complete recoveries. Despite this, these men were censored by the Medical Establishment at the time and were criticized for engaging in what was alleged to be medical quackery.

The argument was, how could respectable doctors advise people with a disease that has a 99 percent mortality rate to ignore all of the established drugs of medical science and go down to the butcher shop and buy some raw liver and take this and expect this to cure a disease that nothing else had cured. Well, raw liver did cure the disease and raw liver prevented it. As the chemistry of raw liver was studied it was discovered that the factors responsible were Vitamin B12[149] and Folic Acid. So Vitamin B12 and Folic Acid are now a part of our normal dietary experience.

And so in 1974, the uninformed, the unimaginative and some of the illiterate are concerned with what to them is a preposterous idea that by eating the seeds of fruit you can

---

[149] Like B17, Vitamin B12 also contains the cyanide radical., hence its name, cyanocobalomin

prevent a disease that carries a mortality rate almost as high as that once carried by pernicious anemia. But scientific truth isn't dependent upon credibility or lack of it. The scientific reality either is or it isn't. And this is the scientific reality - that the seeds of all common fruits (except citrus) contain Vitamin B17, an anti-cancer vitamin. If we ingest proper quantities of this vitamin either in the pure form or through ingesting the nitrilosidic foods, we will be able to prevent this disease just as surely as we are able to prevent scurvy by the use of Vitamin C or pernicious anemia by the use of Vitamin B12.

There was another disease that had a metabolic or chronic nature and this was pellagra. At one time it was so endemic in certain parts of the world, particularly the American South-West, that there were entire hospitals given to the treatment of pellagrins.

The great Sir William Osler in his *Principles and Practices of Medicine*, written at the turn of this century, said of pellagra, *"I was at Lenoir, North Carolina during one winter and I visited the Lenoir home for the colored insane and there 75 percent of the inmates died from the disease. It ran rampant through this institution and convinced me beyond any doubt that pellagra is a virus that is infectious."*

And then came the fine works of the United States Public Health Service surgeon, Dr Goldberger, who showed conclusively that the occurrence of pellagra was related to a deficiency of fresh green material in the diet. So Dr Goldberger approached this problem first by the use of brewer's yeast, which would completely prevent and cure pellagra. Further studies then showed that the factor in brewer's yeast that was most determinate of this effect was niacin, Vitamin B3.

So another fatal chronic metabolic disease found total resolution and cure through factors normal to the regular diet of the animal economy. We know that cancer is no exception to this great generalization which to date has known no exception. That is, that every chronic or metabolic disease that will ever be controlled by man must be controlled by means that are a part of the biological experience of the organism. Chronic and metabolic diseases can never be controlled, prevented or cured by factors [drugs] foreign to the biological experience of the organism.

Dr Thomas of the Sloan-Kettering Institute in a recent article in *Science* said, *"I'm thankful that my liver works without my knowledge. I do not have the brains to commence to do one millionth of what my liver does. These things are automatic. So I swallow the food and this infinitely complex machinery takes care of itself."*

We could spend years telling you about this magnificent machinery and we still wouldn't touch the surface of this infinite ocean. We do know that there is nothing that we can do to improve upon it. We do know that in the history of medicine there never has been found anything foreign to the indwelling requirements of this machinery that will do the living organism any good. And we can go further to say there has never in the history of medicine been found anything foreign to the indwelling machinery of this infinitely complex system that will not harm the organism. There isn't such a thing as a factor foreign to the biological experience that is not harmful to the organism.

There is nothing we can add to our air, water and food to improve it. The most we can do is to look at some of our devitalized food and hopefully attempt to replace that which was capriciously removed from it in the process of food refining, manipulation or cooking. There is absolutely nothing that we can add to that food to improve it. These things are basic.

There isn't any chemical or drug that medical science could suggest that would make us healthier or better adjusted or wiser or give us hope for a longer life. There isn't a single drug or molecule in nature that can accomplish this unless that molecule exists in normal food. And this probably explains one of the reasons why there is so much resistance to laetrile, B17.

The application of this science brings us face to face with a lot of things we do not like to face. We have become over-civilized. We are inclined in our delusory thinking to feel that there must be a magic 'out', that there must be a simple way, a short cut, that somehow or other medical science or some other man-made force beyond our comprehension will do for us those things we must do for ourselves. And it is slowly dawning on us, perhaps too slowly, that this thinking is fraudulent, that it is unsound.

It isn't in the field of cancer alone where we see this form of charlatanism or quackery. We see it in the area of the human mind - the futile attempts to spare man from the realities that surround him. Above all to spare him from the fact that he is accountable to himself and to his God and that there is no short cut in this accountability.

It's real at the physical level. And when we are eating less than adequate food, we know better. And when we continue we are engaged in sin, this is the basis for practically all of our physical and mental and spiritual difficulties. We had better be realistic about it. We have these difficulties because we don't do the right things. And when we fail in view of our knowledge now to take Vitamin B17, this is a sin against our physical nature. And when we develop cancer we will receive the results of this transgression in the old fashion Biblical sense that the "wages of sin are death."

If you are not getting Vitamin B17 in your food, the best way to get it is in the pure form. If you have cancer, the most important single consideration is to get the maximum amount of Vitamin B17 into your body in the shortest period of time. This is secondary to the medical skill involved in administering it, which is relatively minimal. Then very often there are many supportive measures that are taken in the management of the cancer patient such as the use of materials to build up the blood, to raise or lower the blood pressure or to relieve the pain.

Pancreatic enzymes and vegetable enzymes are part of the supportive theory. You have the papaya melons as the source of the enzyme papain and pineapple as a source of the enzyme bromelain. The demasking effect of these enzymes against the pericellular layer of the malignant cell is something very concrete in the immunology of cancer. Now I prefer, rather than advising the use of bromelain or papaya tablets, that the individual seeking these enzymes get them directly from the fresh ripe pineapple and papaya fruit. As much as half a pineapple a day should be ingested.

This is the way to go. You have nothing to lose by eating fresh pineapple and papaya melons. Nothing to lose by eating millet, the seeds of all the common fruits and whole fresh foods.

Dietary deficiencies arrive primarily from eating less than whole food. This is why the American federal and state governments have made mandatory the artificial enrichment of white flour. Look at any loaf of white bread or white flour that has been enriched by the addition of crystalline Vitamin B1, Vitamin B2, niacin, iron and all the rest. What a commentary on the stupidity of our civilization that we put good food through a process that deprives it of its essential nutrients and then we are compelled by government mandate to restore to this food some of the things that have been processed out. One of the most critical factors is removed and that is wheat germ, which contains the

135

Vitamin E and the polyunsaturated fatty acids. It would not be necessary to take it in supplementation if our foods were not manipulated in a way which removes these factors.

Now something about supplementation in addition to the Vitamin B17. We can't think in terms of just one vitamin. We get an adequate diet by eating as wide a variety of whole natural foods as possible and as close to their growing period as we can possibly obtain them.

There are laetrile therapists who recommend two or three grams of ascorbic acid or Vitamin C in conjunction with the laetrile program. This is a very moderate recommendation and we can all take up to seven or eight grams of Vitamin C without any problems. This is about the same amount as animals such as the gorilla, on a pound-to-pound basis, ingest - between five to six grams of Vitamin C a day in their normal habitat. Incidentally, the gorilla in its natural habitat eats about 100 to 125 milligrams of Vitamin B17 every day too. Like the population of Hunzaland, these gorillas are free of cancer.

Bears are also free of cancer in their normal habitat. In the wild, bears don't develop cancer. In the San Diego Zoo, there was a cage of about ten bears and out of the ten, seven of them developed cancer. To some this was a sign that some mysterious bear cancer virus was loose, but it wasn't that at all. In the wild state, bears are omnivores and they eat a lot of wild nitrilosidic berries. Almost all wild fruits are nitrilosidic.

Keep in mind how far we have drifted from the dietary requirements of the machinery we possess. The fruit we eat today is the product of years of manipulation and cultivation for lushness and abundance and so forth, so the meat to that fruit is free of Vitamin B17. To meet our indwelling needs of Vitamin B17 we must either eat the fruit seed in reasonable quantities or begin supplementing our diet with

Vitamin B17 tablets. We can't of course do that at present [due to legislation], but we hope to see before very long Vitamin B17 available so that we can prevent cancer in the same way we prevent scurvy.

Several new books are coming out on laetrile. Both are written by non-medical men: *World Without Cancer* by Edward Griffin and *Vitamin B17: Forbidden Weapon Against Cancer* by Mike Culbert. We are all laymen in the field of cancer. There are laymen in the laetrile movement who know more about cancer than some of our most prestigious experts in our most prestigious institutions. These laymen know enough about it to keep alive and not die from it. So you're a pretty rotten expert if you know so little about it as to succumb from it or have your family succumb from it.

We have many case histories of people that have been helped by laetrile. Both Alicia Buttons and Mary Henderson were terminal with oral pharyngeal cancer that has a mortality rate of 98-99 percent even in early diagnosis. Both made remarkable recoveries with laetrile under the guidance of Dr Hans Nieper in Germany.

You know we have been meeting for ten or eleven years and you've been hearing this story. Each time after the meeting you had 360 days to go home and read newspapers, American Cancer Society technical journals, Boiler Plate and so forth. In those ten years they haven't told you anything against laetrile that makes any sense. You can be pretty sure they don't have anything against laetrile because these people are very uninhibited and the area in which they are most uninhibited is the area of simple lying.

If you have any questions about laetrile, the more critical the better because we are dealing with solid science. We are dealing with a science that admits that there is no rational alternative in the ten years that have passed since these meetings began. Nothing has come about which does anything except make more obvious the fact that laetrile, Vitamin B17, is the answer to cancer."

FAQ
Frequently Asked Questions

Q: What are the long-term survival prospects for cancer sufferers who treat their illness with B17 Metabolic Therapy?

A: Survival prospects of any kind for those taking B17/Metabolic Therapy depend on the extent to which the patient's immune system and organs have been weakened by the effects of orthodox therapies, such as drugs, x-rays or other immuno-suppressant activity. The problem is, most newly diagnosed patients don't opt for vitamin therapy to start with because of the bias of cancer specialists towards persuading their patients to undergo conventional, allopathic treatment. Consequently a high percentage of those who end up taking metabolic (vitamin) therapies do so as a last resort after being sent home by their doctors with a hopeless prognosis. That any should survive at all with B17 and its complementary therapies at this point is a miracle in itself.

Edward Griffin reports in his book that on average, long-term survival (over five years) can be expected in 15% of cases where the cancer has metastasised, if these are treated with B17 as the primary therapy. This figure is in comparison to only one case in one thousand surviving long-term for metastatic patients treated with orthodox therapies.[150]

In cases where cancer is first diagnosed, long-term survival for vitamin therapy is gauged at around 80% as compared with 28% for orthodox therapies. Long-term prevention from cancer using a detoxifying high plant dietary and adequate supplies of B17 in the diet, together with a clean, non-carcinogenic environment (there are things we can change, and things we can't in this regard) is as close to 100% as you can get. A control group for this prevention study already exists with the Hunzakuts, Abkhasians, the Eskimos, Hopi Indians and similar populations around the world.

---

[150] See also **Binzel MD, Philip** *Alive and Well.....* available through Credence Publications at www.credence.org.

One must understand that there are many factors affecting the outcome of a cancer and there is no guarantee of a recovery from cancer with nutritional therapy. The above statistics are very approximate and do vary according to age, sex, cancer location, level of malignancy, length and type of treatment. Fortunately enough data has been compiled by Drs. Krebs, Richardson, Contreras, Nieper, Sugiura, Burk and others to give orthodox treatments every conceivable advantage in the reckoning. Nevertheless, B17 still demonstrates benefits for survivability and recovery far beyond those attained with orthodox therapies. The data for nutrition as a highly effective treatment for cancer is simply too impressive to brush aside.

Q: Does Metabolic Therapy cure ALL cancers?

A: Those who prescribe Metabolic Therapy are careful to state that B17 does not 'cure' cancer but appears to be the control and preventative for the disease. A cure suggests that once the disease has been defeated, one can cease taking the curative. This however is NOT the case with metabolic deficiency diseases, such as scurvy and pellagra. If we accept that cancer is a chronic, metabolic deficiency disease, then B17 may be viewed as the missing component which can restore nutritional balance to the organism. The rest of the nutritional program centres on ridding the patient of toxins accumulated in their system over the years and restoring adequate levels of pancreatic enzymes through a drastic reduction of animal proteins in the diet.

Once cancer is regressed or even eliminated, B17 must, for the remaining life of the patient, be maintained in adequate supplies in the diet of the subject. Just as with scurvy, if the vitamin component is subsequently removed, the disease will certainly return.

With that in mind, a wide range of cancers has been reported to respond very favourably to the combined metabolic protocol. Lung cancer, pancreatic cancer, liver, brain, leukaemia, lymph, bone, testicular, prostate, skin, breast, uterine, cervical, colorectal, etc. As time progresses and medicine becomes more accepting of nutritional treatments for cancer, a wider range of data will be amassed. Internet sites operated by doctors practising Metabolic Therapy are a great source of information for individual case testimonies and details of treatments. Please see the Internet references listed in this book.

Q: Who are some of the top doctors who have embraced Metabolic Therapy and the deficiency concept of cancer?

A: Some of the many are as follows:

West Germany: Dr Hans Nieper, former Director of the Department of Medicine at Silbersee Hospital in Hanover. Pioneered cobalt therapy and the anti-cancer drug *cyclophosphamide*. Former head of Aschaffenburg Hospital Laboratory. Listed in *Who's Who in World Science*. Former Director of the German Society for Medical Tumour Treatment. During a visit to the United States in 1972, Dr Nieper told reporters: *"After more than twenty years of such specialised work, I have found non-toxic nitrilosides – that is, laetrile – far superior to any other known cancer treatment or preventative. In my opinion, it is the only existing possibility for the ultimate control of cancer."*

Canada: Dr N R Bouziane, former Director of Research Laboratories at St Jeanne D'Arc Hospital in Montreal. Dean of the merican Association of Bio-Analysts. He also received a doctorate in science from the University of Montreal and St Joseph's University, an affiliate of Oxford University in New Brunswick. Dr Bouziane's repeated successes in treating cancers with laetrile were written up in the *Cancer News Journal*, Jan/April 1971, p.20 under the article heading "The Laetrile Story".

Philippines: Dr Manuel Navarro, former Professor of Medicine and Surgery at the University of Santo Tomas, Manila. Associate Member of the National Research Council of the Philippines. A Fellow of the Philippine College of Physicians, the Philippine Society of Endocrinology and Metabolism. A member of the Philippine Medical Association, the Philippine Cancer Society and many other medical groups. Dr Navarro is an internationally recognised cancer researcher with over 100 major scientific papers to his credit, some read before the International Cancer Congress. Dr Navarro has treated terminally ill cancer patients with laetrile for over 25 years. He stated in the *Cancer News Journal*: *"It is my carefully considered clinical judgement, as a practising oncologist and researcher in this field, that I have obtained most significant and encouraging results with the use of laetrile-amygdalin in the treatment of terminal cancer patients...*[151]*"*

Mexico: Dr Ernesto Contreras, one of Mexico's leading medical specialists, has operated the Oasis Hospital in Tijuana, Mexico for over 30 years, treating cancer patients with laetrile. Many of his patients have travelled from America where laetrile treatment is currently denied them by law. Dr Contreras received post-graduate training at the Harvard Children's Hospital in Boston. He has served as the chief pathologist at the Army Hospital in Mexico City and was Professor of Histology and Pathology at the Mexican Army Medical School.

Dr Contreras remarks of B17-laetrile's action with extreme terminal cancer cases: *"The palliative action* [the ability of a substance to improve the comfort of a patient] *is in about 60% of the cases. Frequently, enough to be significant, I see arrest of the disease or even regression in some 15% of the very advanced cases*[152]*."*

Italy: Professor Etore Guidetti of the University of Turin Medical School. Dr Guidetti addressed the Conference of the International Union Against Cancer held in Brazil in 1954 and announced startling results with laetrile in successfully combating many types of cancer, including cervix, breast, uterus and rectum. After his speech, an American doctor rose in the audience, challenging the Italian professor that laetrile had been found to be worthless in the United States. Dr Guidetti was abrupt and dismissive: *"I care not*

---

[151] *Cancer News Journal,* Jan/April 1971, pp.19-21

[152] These are cases receiving a 100% death-rate prognosis, given up as hopeless by orthodox medicine. The fact that any of these survive *at all* is astonishing in itself. Dr Contreras' words were reported in the *Cancer News Journal*, ibid.

what was determined in the United States. I am merely reporting what I saw in my own clinic[153]."

Belgium: Professor Joseph H Maisin, Sr from the University of Louvain, Director of the Institute of Cancer. Professor Maisin was also President Emeritus of the International League Against Cancer which holds the International Cancer Congress every four years.

United States: Among the many, Dr Ernst T Krebs Jr, who developed laetrile. Dr Harold W Manner, professor of biology, Loyola University, Chicago. Dr H Ray Evers, Dr Dan Dotson and Dr John A Richardson of Albany, California. Dr John A Morrone of the Jersey City Medical Center. 60-year cancer researcher Dr Kanematsu Sugiura of Memorial Sloan-Kettering, and Dr Dean Burk, a founding member of the American National Cancer Institute and head of its Cytochemistry Section. Dr Burk was also recipient of the Gerhard Domagk Award for Cancer Research, the Hillebrand Award of the American Chemical Society, Fellow of the National Research Council at the University of London, of the Kaiser Wilhelm Institute for Biology and also Harvard. Dr Burk belonged to eleven scientific organisations, published over two hundred scientific papers in the field of cell chemistry and authored three books on cancer research.

Q: How do you respond to charges by the medical establishment that laetrile proponents cannot produce one substantiated case which shows any shred of evidence for B17 having a positive effect against cancer?

A: Gasp! As of 1976, there were upwards of 6,000 'shreds of evidence' from the caseload of Dr John A Richardson. A carefully researched 4,800 cases by Mexico's Dr Ernesto Contreras (culled from some 10,000 medical records developed by him in 14 years experience with Laetrile - as of the year 2000, over 100,000 patients). Almost 4,000 cases of total metabolic treatment by Dr E Paul Wedel of Oregon, himself a Laetrile recovery patient. 1,000 cases documented by Dr Manuel D Navarro, University of Santo

---

[153] *Cancer News Journal*, ibid.

Tomas, Manila, Philippines. A cluster of 100 Mexican government-monitored cases under the guidance of Dr Mario Soto de Leon, medical director at the new Cydel Clinic, Tijuana, Mexico. And then there are the additional thousands treated by Dr Hans Nieper, West Germany and thousands more treated by a group of Laetrile-using physicians in the United States, including the records of Dr Philip Binzel, and such cancer victims as Glen Rutherford, Kansas, whose total recovery by Laetrile therapy at Tijuana is described in court records as a "cure."

Q: The book seems to deal with the story of nutritional therapy from an American point of view. Has there been a similar controversy in England?
A: Good question. The answer appears to be no. Our research team contacted the Medicines Control Agency in Vauxhall, London to determine their attitude towards laetrile. We received a very polite reply from a spokesman who advised us that laetrile was not used in England, but that if ever it were to be, the substance would be subject to the MCA's drug regulatory process because laetrile contains cyanide. Naturally therefore their spokesman knows something of laetrile and its chemistry. Personally I don't believe the MCA is as ignorant of the situation as they're letting on. Top marks for politeness though.

An article printed in the *Express*, *Telegraph* and *The Week* reported that Professor Monica Hughes of Newcastle University had experienced success in treating a brain tumour in a rat using cyanide released from the tropical plant cassava[154]. I telephoned Professor Hughes and asked her if she was aware of laetrile. After jogging her memory she replied that she had heard through the press (probably the MacDonald/Garland report) that it was a hoax. Once again, her opinion was formed from propaganda rather than the facts, ironically even in the face of the fact that Professor

---

[154] *Daily Telegraph*, 13th April 1999; *The Week*, 10th April 1999

Hughes' cyanide from cassava is merely the B17 in this robust, nitrilosidic plant![155]

Interestingly drug companies are attempting to synthesise the cyanide release system of B17, presumably with patents and £300 capsules in mind. At the bottom of *The Week* article, the last sentence reads, *"A drug company is now looking into whether the process could work in humans."* This is pretty sad considering that knowledge of selective cyanide releasing at cancer sites has been part of general medical understanding for the better part of 50 years. As we've just seen, even the *Cancer News Journal* was writing about laetrile back in the early 70s.

Q: I appreciate that, as a non-medical researcher, you cannot dispense medical advice. But what immediate steps would YOU take if you contracted cancer, based on what you have found out?
A: What would I do? That's easy. I would immediately commence Phase 1 Metabolic Therapy and supplement this with 25 apricot seeds a day and key Neways supplements such as Maximol, Cascading Revenol, Hawaiian Noni, the parasite cleanser Purge and Cassie-Tea. During the entire treatment process, I would be eating 90% unrefined plant dietary in the form of fruit only in the morning and then properly combined natural foods to detoxify my organism. Phase 2 would follow 21 days later for a further three months. I would ingest 7g of Vitamin C a day[156] and consume papayas and half a pineapple each morning during the fruit intake for additional supplies of enzymes such as papain and bromelain (these enzymes are also available in capsule form in Phases 1 & 2). I would remove as many toxins as possible from my food, such as caffeine, refined sugars and additives. I would commence a healthy diet of fruit and vegetables to detoxify and de-

---

[155] According to FDA toxicologist June de Spain, the tropical plant cassava is rich in Vitamin B17 (*The Little Cyanide Cookbook*, ibid).
[156] Controversial Vitamin C pioneer Dr Linus Pauling maintained that cancer sufferers should ingest up to 10g of this vitamin each day for optimum protection against the disease. Dr Pauling was derided for making such statements, but outlived all of his detractors, enjoying paramount health and working long hours on horseback on his ranch in Big Sur, California up to within a few weeks of his death at age 94.

stress my organism. I would cut out meat and commence eating lightly broiled fish rich in essential vitamins and oils. I would reject all orthodox cancer treatments from the outset, including exploratory surgical biopsies (also mammograms for females). Instead I would elect to have a hCG urine test, 95% accurate in testing for cancer trophoblast. I would only consider surgery an option if my tumours were immediately life-threatening (this is not usually the case when cancer is initially diagnosed)[157].

Cancer is no light matter and a qualified medical practitioner should always be consulted when undergoing even nutritional therapy. One has to understand the principles of vitamin treatment, why it works and how it works, and then go for it 'by the book'. Education in this matter is so important. There are many who dip their toes into Metabolic Therapy but who do not 'own' the treatment and carry it out the way the professionals have recommended. I encourage everyone NOW to research this subject thoroughly. Now is the safe time, before cancer starts, to learn about the options and most importantly, to exercise prevention. These are the acceptable days. How much better not to have to worry about cancer in the first place.

Q: Prevention: How do I NOT get cancer in the first place?

A: Dr Ernst Krebs and others state that wholesome foods (70-80% unrefined plant dietary and low meat intakes), excellent supplementary nutrition (full nutritional supplementation including ionised minerals and high quality antioxidants) and 10 apricot kernels per day for life will ensure that you will never have to deal with cancer. I believe them. Krebs wanted everyone chewing 10 seeds each day. There is also the environmental toxin side of the equation that needs to be addressed. You should clear the obvious cancer dangers from your life that are known to be problems, such as smoking, stress and a poor, additive- and meat-heavy diet. Meat, especially beef, can contain estrogen additives such as Estradiol to fatten the animals. Meat-eating promotes estrogens in the body, causing a higher risk of trophoblast triggering. Meat, as

---

[157] See section entitled *What is Metabolic Therapy?*

we have also seen, is responsible for depleting supplies of pancreatic enzymes in the body.

Existing personal and household care products should also be exchanged for safe, non-carcinogenic alternatives. Do it today. Neways is the company to use to accomplish this and details on how to obtain these products are given in the section entitled *Contacts! Contacts! Contacts!* It's a transfer spend, so you won't be paying out loads of additional money to 'live safe'.

Q: Can nutritional therapy be successfully used alongside orthodox treatments?

A: Doctors experienced in treating cancer patients with Metabolic Therapy indicate that chemotherapy and radiotherapy, while appearing to reduce tumour size, have a traumatising effect on the body in general and even in certain cases help metastasise the cancer by weakening the patient's immune system. There never has been any evidence that these orthodox treatments in any way extend the life of the patient over the long haul in the common epithelial cancers. Often we see the complete opposite. With chemotherapy, indiscriminate cell poisoning IS the object, and thus we see patients becoming gravely ill from the treatments themselves. A tragic case in point involved US Senator Paul Tsongas, who died in hospital in January 1997. His obituary stated: *"Hospitalized Jan 3 with a liver problem because of cancer treatments. Tsongas was cancer-free at his death."*

In a letter from Dr John A Richardson to Edward Griffin dated 2nd December 1972, Dr Richardson stated: *"I have seen patients who have been paralyzed by cobalt spine radiation, and after vitamin treatment their hCG test is faintly positive. We got their cancer, but the radiogenic manipulation is such that they can't walk... It's the cobalt that will kill, not the cancer."*

The answer to the question therefore is that Metabolic Therapy will work alongside orthodox treatments if it has to. It will even mitigate some of the collateral effects of toxicity from these treatments. But its efficacy will be reduced due to organ damage and impairment of the patient's liver and immune system brought on by the toxicity and radiation of the orthodox treatments.

Q: I've heard that apple seeds are good for you but toxic in extremely large quantities. Is this true?

A: That's perfectly true. Once again the apple seed is rich in B17, containing hydrogen cyanide and benzaldehyde. There was an unsubstantiated story of a person who quaffed a whole bucket of apple seeds and went down with cyanide poisoning. Firstly, anyone who eats a bucket of apple seeds is too stupid to live. Secondly, this was an unsubstantiated story – one of a few – no doubt designed to bring on doubt in the minds of the public as to the effectiveness of nutritional therapy.

Let's exercise a little common sense. Too much of anything is going to put you in harm's way. In the case of B17, the enzyme rhodanese detoxifies the unwanted hydrocyanic acid into by-products, which actually nourish healthy tissue. But please note this: If the ingestion of B17 exceeds the rate at which our bodies can break down the surplus, then of course there is going to be a problem. Excess will always be a problem. After all, drink too much water and you'll drown.

A good rule of thumb for cancer prevention and one that allows plenty of margin for safety is this: Do not eat more of the seeds than you would eat of the fruit. If you are clinically cancerous, then a different regimen is advised by the clinics, as outlined by some of the practitioners quoted in this book. You have nothing to fear from B17, in spite of all the twaddle being bandied about. Just get educated on the subject and be wise.

Q: Does B17 work for dogs, cats and other animals suffering from cancer?

A: I hear tales all the time. There are several B17 testimonies for animals at http://www.apricotsfromgod.com/journal. I always have folks coming up to me at the seminars and telling me the good news of what happened to Fifi, when everyone though that she was lost. Just as with the mice we heard about earlier, all animal systems are capable of responding to Metabolic Therapy. Wild animals don't get cancer because they have ready access to natural foods rich in nitrilosides. It is only when these animals are fed diets by modern man that some develop problems with cancer because the B17 element goes missing.

Q: Yeetchh! I hate the taste of apricot seeds. Can I swallow them whole?

A: The best medicine always tastes the worst! Actually I really like the taste. The best way to eat the seeds is to crunch them in the mouth, massage the bits into a saliva paste and allow the taste to infuse the tissue of the mouth. After chewing for a while, the pulp may then be swallowed. This is said to be the best way to ensure a full B17 assimilation. So, go ahead, pinch your nose, don't be a baby and go for it! They actually compliment the taste of the fruit you eat them with too.

Do not swallow these seeds whole. Firstly, you will not benefit from their nutrition and secondly, you will need the services of Dyno-Rod to unblock your plumbing! Those who really have a problem with the taste may grind up the seeds and use them as a spice for their food. An excellent book, *The Little Cyanide Cookbook* by June de Spain (available through Credence), can also be purchased for hundreds of recipes which include apricot seeds and other nitrilosidic foods in every imaginable disguise. June actually worked for the FDA as a toxicologist and so is eminently qualified to write such a book.

But please be advised, so me have stopped taking the seeds because of the taste, believing that the B17 tablets are sufficient in themselves for treatment of clinical cancer. All the evidence shows that it is a combination of the two treatments, seeds and B17, along with complementary therapies such as Vitamins A, E & C, Cassie-Tea, bromelain/chymotrypsin enzymes and full nutritional support with Maximol and Revenol that is the most effective. This regimen must be practised along with the requisite changes in diet: Fruit alone in the morning; drastically reduce meats and animal proteins, and properly combine proteins and carbohydrates (see section entitled: *What is Metabolic Therapy?*)

Q: How do you respond to accusations that B17 is just another 'snake-oil' cancer remedy that falsely raises hopes, milks the sick and desperate of their money and can in fact be dangerous in the form of apricot seeds?

A: Recently a hostile oncologist raised this very point with me regarding the supposed toxicity of standard doses of B17. Aside from pointing out to this man that I take my medicine daily whereas he doesn't and routinely prescribes chemotherapy drugs of EXTREME toxicity to many of his patients, I asked him why we shouldn't set up a little practical demonstration wherein he took his cancer medicine for two months and I'd take mine. Then at the end, we could see whose therapies were the most dangerous. He angrily hung up the telephone. Folks, I've eaten apple and peach seeds for years, and these days consume 60+ apricot seeds a day, not because I am proving a point, but because I love 'em. And I'm still here!

Regarding the 'snake-oil' point, those challenging B17 on this basis are presumably completely ignorant of the calibre of medicinal science that has already validated laetrile/amygdalin and used it very successfully as a cancer treatment procedure for humans and animals for over three decades. We have dealt with some of these points in the book. Edward Griffin does a fuller job in his title. In the end, scoffers will always scoff. People have been scoffing at nutritional therapy for forty years but it still heals cancer.

What is Metabolic Therapy?

Please note: The following information is compiled from treatments carried out by some cancer clinics around the world. These treatments are widely believed by many in the alternative cancer treatment field to be most effective in combating cancers and/or acting as strong cancer preventatives in human and animal systems. No claims are made or implied in providing the following information. The reader must use his discretion and a qualified medical practitioner should always be consulted in the matter of treatment decisions for any cancer.

"If you have cancer, the most important single consideration is to get the maximum amount of Vitamin B17 into your body in the shortest period of time. This is secondary to the medical skill involved in administering it, which is relatively minimal." – Ernst T Krebs Jr

"Metabolic Therapy, put simply, is the use of natural food products and vitamins to prevent and treat cancer by building a strong immune system. The key to stopping the cancer growth doesn't lie in traditional cancer treatments like chemo and radiation therapy or surgery, but in an approach that works with the body instead of against it.

Once the body is cleansed of unnatural substances (detoxification) and vitamins are administered to build the immune system, enzymes are given to begin breaking down the protein shell which surrounds the cancer growth and protects it from the body's immune system. Raw glandular products are also used to augment the body's natural glands. Vitamin B17 (laetrile) and Vitamin A are then given to the patient to work with the enzymes and immune system to destroy the cancer cell.

Initially laetrile was looked upon as useless, which it is when used in isolation. However, in Metabolic Therapy, it works with enzymes, vitamins and the immune system to destroy the already weakened cancer." – Dr Harold W Manner

Nutritional therapy for cancer is endorsed by many doctors, including Drs Ernesto and Francisco Contreras, two of the world's most famous and successful cancer physicians. The Contreras Research Team has investigated more than 75 different therapies for cancer in the past 34 years and treated over 100,000 patients. The team continues to seek out the most advanced, effective and compassionate treatments in the world.

B17 METABOLIC THERAPY OVERVIEW
(Phase 1 - The First 21 Days)

The initial phase consists of a 21-day therapy in which clinics include an intravenous drip of B17, sometimes combined with the tissue-penetrating agent DMSO and high doses of Vitamin C. However 500mg amygdalin tablets, together with apricot kernels, are often employed for home use if intravenous treatment is not available. Supplementary therapies in Phase 1 include pancreatic enzyme formula, Vitamin C (up to 10g/day), antioxidants, such as Cascading Revenol, Vitamins A & E (emulsion), BarleyGreen powder, shark cartilage (100% pure), and actual whole foods that contain B17 (e.g. apricot seeds). Detoxification and full nutritional supplementation procedures are also rigorously followed.

B17 METABOLIC THERAPY
(Phase 2 - The Next 3 Months)

The second phase consists of Vitamin B17/amygdalin tablets, apricot seeds, enzymes, Vitamins A, C and E, shark cartilage and the continuing detoxification and nutritional procedures initiated in Phase 1.

COMBINED MODALITIES OF TREATMENT

There are no contraindications using amygdalin or any of the components of Metabolic Therapy along with surgery, radiation and chemotherapy, according to the clinics. Surgery, for example, is often life-saving with cancer patients by correcting blockages, repairing fistulas, arresting haemorrhages and removing cancerous growths that are threatening vital organs. If surgery can remove a tumour completely, as in early, non-metastatic cancer, it may conserve the health and save the life of the patient.

What's In Metabolic Therapy?

Phase 1 Metabolic Pack for the first 21 days

Comes in two alternative forms:

PHASE 1 INTRAVENOUS

With injectable B17/Amygdalin ampoules for administration by qualified medical practitioner. This pack comprises:

- Vitamin B17 ampoules
- Cascading Revenol capsules (contains powerful antioxidants)
- Pancreatic enzyme tablets
- Vitamin C
- Vitamin A & E emulsion drops
- Maximol Solutions (colloidal mineral supplement)
- Hawaiian Noni Juice (anti-tumoural)

Not included is DMSO (dimethyl sulfoxide) for IV administration (some doctors use this compound to achieve fuller penetration of the B17) and apricot kernels.

OR

PHASE 1 ORAL

Injectable/IV Amygdalin is replaced with 500mg Amygdalin tablets. Otherwise the ORAL Phase 1 includes the same materials as above. Can be purchased for home use. Not included are apricot kernels for nutritional support.

Then, after the first 21 days….

PHASE 2 for the next 3 months

Pack comprises B17 in 500mg tablet form with the same materials as Phase 1. Not included are apricot kernels for nutritional support.

NUTRITIONAL THERAPY COMPONENT DESCRIPTIONS
(Advanced nutritional elements and their modality)

The following section, compiled by this author and other contributors, outlines nutritional components that have been studied and used for specific purposes in relation to nutritional support for those who have

153

cancer or those wishing to exercise prevention. The purpose of this section is to inform and not to recommend any particular course of action. Health advice from a qualified health practitioner trained in nutrition is always advised.

Injectable B17/Laetrile/Amygdalin

Pharmaceutical grade Vitamin B17 in Metabolic Therapy clinics is administered through injection for the first 21 days (Phase 1) and then orally afterwards (Phase 2). 9 grams per day is used for the first 21 days in Del Rio Hospital. Dr Manner used this protocol. Injectable B17 is also invariably administered together with the tissue penetrating agent dimethylsulfoxide (DMSO) (see DMSO section).

Please note: Clinical tests have repeatedly shown that B17 is only truly effective when used in conjunction with pancreatic enzymes to break down the pericellular coating of the malignant cell[158]. Vitamins A and E in their emulsified form, along with high doses of Vitamin C, are then used in combination with B17 to attack the cancer cell. Clinics administering Metabolic Therapy to their patients always use these or similar supplements.

B17 Laetrile/Amygdalin Tablets

These pharmaceutical grade tablets contain the active B17 ingredient derived from the kernels of apricots. Usually available in 100mg or 500mg tablets. Some people are confused with the terms laetrile and amygdalin. These names essentially refer to the same compound – Vitamin B17 – and are, to all intents and purposes, interchangeable. These tablets are always taken in conjunction with the apricot seeds. Manufacturers recommend:

---

[158] **Manner, HW, Michaelson, TL, and DiSanti, SJ**. "Enzymatic Analysis of Normal and Malignant Tissues." Presented at the Illinois State Academy of Science, April 1978. Also Manner, HW, Michaelson, TL, and DiSanti, SJ, "Amygdalin, Vitamin A and Enzymes Induced Regression of Murine Mammary Adenocarcinomas", *Journal of Manipulative and Physiological Therapeutics*, Vol 1, No. 4, December 1978. 200 East Roosevelt Road, Lombard, IL 60148 USA

- 2-4 100mg tablets per day as a nutritional supplement for prevention (apricot seeds have been recommended by doctors in place of tablets for prevention also).
- 4-6 500mg tablets per day as a nutritional supplement for clinical cancer sufferers, taken in conjunction with enzymes and Vitamins A & E (emulsified). Cascading Revenol is also sometimes used in place of Vitamin A (emulsified).

Pancreatic Enzyme Supplements

Specific enzymes used in Metabolic Therapy include chymotrypsin (human pancreatic enzyme), pancreatin and calf thymus (animal enzymes), papain (from papayas) and bromelain (from pineapples). Ernst Krebs also states: *"The demasking effect of these enzymes against the pericellular layer of the malignant cell is something very concrete in the immunology of cancer. Now I prefer, rather than advising the use of bromelain or papaya tablets, that the individual seeking these enzymes get them directly from the fresh ripe pineapple and papaya fruit. As much as half a pineapple a day should be ingested."*

Emulsified Vitamin A

In 1963 when Dr Contreras initiated his activities as a clinical oncologist, the use of Vitamin A as a useful agent in malignant neoplasm was considered illogical and absurd. Now Vitamin A is accepted as an agent of great use for the major epithelial cancers as well as for epidermis carcinomas, chronic leukaemia and transitional cells.

The first formal studies of the possible anti-tumour effects of Vitamin A were initiated in Germany, by investigators of Mugos Laboratories in Munich. It was a proven fact that lung cancer in Norwegian sailors was less common than in other groups, even though they smoked since childhood. Logic indicated that it had to be the opposite. After studying this phenomenon, it was discovered that they ate abundant quantities of raw fish liver, high in Vitamin A, since childhood. The logical conclusion was that high doses of such a vitamin prevented the growth of lung cancer in heavy smokers. But it was also found that high doses of Vitamin A were toxic, and could cause adverse reactions.

The main focus was to find out how to administer enough Vitamin A to observe preventive or healing effects, without injuring the liver. The solution was found by one of the investigators, when he discovered that unprocessed milk had the vitamin, and children who were breast-fed never experienced toxic effects. Nature had the solution by including Vitamin A in milk in the form of micro-emulsification.

Mugos investigators proceeded to prepare a variety of emulsified concentrations, formulating their famous High Concentration A-Mulsin. One drop contains 15,000 units. They were able to administer over a million units per day in progressive doses, without producing hepatic toxicity. The explanation is that, in emulsified form, Vitamin A is absorbed directly into the lymphatic system without going through the liver in high quantities. Having solved the toxicity problem, it was possible to test the product in high doses. It was demonstrated that emulsified Vitamin A has the following effects:

- In normal doses, it protects epithelium and vision.
- In doses of 100,000 to 300,000 units per day, it works as a potent immune stimulant.
- In doses of 500,000 to 1,000,000 units per day, it works as a potent anti-tumour agent, especially in epidermis and transitional carcinomas.

Shark Cartilage
It has been said that sharks are the healthiest beings on earth. Sharks are immune to practically every disease known to man. Many scientists believe that the shark's skeleton, composed entirely of cartilage, is what is responsible for its incredible immunity to disease.

When administered to cancer patients, shark cartilage has been reported to inhibit the growth of blood vessels, thereby restricting the vitality of the cancerous tumour. In addition, shark cartilage stimulates the production of antibodies and boosts the immune system. Not only is this a non-toxic product recommended for the treatment of cancer, but also for the treatment of inflammatory diseases such as rheumatism and osteoarthritis. Tumours are reported frequently to experience significant reduction in size within one to three months of the initial treatment. It is also noted to enhance the efficacy of Vitamin B17/amygdalin. For in-depth information about shark cartilage, *Jaws of Life* by Dr Alex Duarte and *Sharks Don't Get Cancer* by Dr William Lane provide the complete story. Shark cartilage may be contra-indicated with pregnant or lactating women.

Apricot Seeds/Kernels

Apricot kernels are an inexpensive, rich and natural source of Vitamin B17. They also deliver the vitamins, minerals and enzymes not found in the pharmaceutical derivative of B17.

- ❑ 10 seeds per day for life are recommended by Dr Krebs as a nutritional supplement for those exercising cancer prevention.
- ❑ 30-50 seeds per day are recommended by Dr Krebs as nutritional support for clinical cancer sufferers.

In a minority of cases, cancer sufferers may experience nausea when taking seeds. In this event, clinics recommend that dosage is reduced and then gradually increased as tolerance is gained. Not all apricot seeds are effective. They must have the characteristic bitter taste indicating that the active B17 ingredient is present. Not to be eaten whole. May be pulped, grated or crushed.

Please note: Some cancer sufferers believe that apricot kernels alone are all that is required to fight cancer. Consultation with a qualified health practitioner familiar with Metabolic Therapy is advised for further information. Apricot kernels are usually part of the nutritional support for those exercising cancer prevention *for life* as well as cancer patients undergoing Phase 1 or Phase 2 Metabolic Therapy.

Maximol (Neways International)

The huge rise in incidences of cancer and other degenerative diseases are primarily due to the depleted vitamin/mineral content in today's western diet coupled with environmental/chemical toxin factors. The key nutritional ingredients invariably missing for cancer are B17 and the trace mineral selenium. A recent US study showed an overall drop of 50% in cancer deaths and a fall of 37% in new cancer cases, especially lung, bowel and prostate – among 1,300 volunteers taking supplements for four years[159].

Mineral supplementation is most effective in the ionised 'liquid suspension' form, assisted by fulvic acid, where a 98% assimilation by the body is expected, as against 48% for chelated minerals and 10-12% for metallic minerals. Our bodies use minerals as raw material. These cannot be manufactured by the body and so have to be present in the food and liquids we ingest. Sadly, as mentioned previously, our food chain is severely depleted of minerals, resulting in over 150 nutritional deficiency diseases that are now striking our societies with increasing intensity.

To combat this very real threat, mineral and vitamin supplementation, far from being a quaint health fad, is essential for everyone and can literally make the difference between life or death, especially for those with cancer. To combat this threat, Neways has formulated Maximol Solutions, probably the world's most complete liquid nutritional supplement, which contains 67 essential and trace minerals, 17 essential vitamins, 21 amino acids, three enzymes, and lactobacillus acidophilus. To provide greater absorption of all these ingredients, Maximol has been formulated with nature's natural chelator, used by plants and animals for the absorption of minerals and nutrients - organic fulvic acid. It is known that fulvic acid aids in the transport and assimilation of minerals and nutrients into living cells. This may in part be due to its low molecular weight, its electrical potential, and its bio-transporting ability. Fulvic acid aids in the selective trading or supply of minerals and other nutrient factors inside the cell. Fulvic acid is effective at neutralising a wide range of toxic material - from heavy metals and radioactive waste to petrochemicals.

---

[159] *Daily Mail*, 28th July 1999, p. 31

Before minerals can be utilised, they must first be converted from their particular colloidal state to a micro-colloidal state. Thus, for greater bio-availability, Neways has formulated Maximol Solutions as an organic fulvic acid complexed micro-colloidal solution. In this form, Maximol provides higher percentages of easily assimilated minerals than non-ionised colloidal mineral supplements, whose particles are often too large for easy absorption.

Revenol (Neways International)

Scientists tell us that vitamins A, C, and E, as well as beta carotene and other antioxidant bioflavonoids, are vitally important to good health. But there are antioxidant formulae around now that have many more times the power of Vitamin C and Vitamin E. The Neways product Revenol contains antioxidants that are broad-spectrum. Revenol contains antioxidants from maritime pine bark and grape seed pycnogenols extracts - up to 95% in concentration and bioavailability. Revenol also contains curcuminoids – nature's most powerful and aggressive antioxidant, which is around 150 times more powerful than Vitamin E, about 60 times more powerful than Vitamin C, and about 3 times more powerful than antioxidants from maritime pine bark and grape seed pycnogenols extract[160].

Revenol also contains ginkgo biloba for the brain and circulatory system; alpha and beta carotene to increase potency; Esterfied Vitamin C - a bonded form of Vitamin C that increases its power and residual retention in the body (up to 3 days); natural Vitamin E for greater absorption and effectiveness. Micro-spheres are also included which bond to the intestinal wall, allowing up to 400% more of the ingredients to be digested and absorbed.

Each tablet of Revenol supplies over 60 milligrams of curcuminoids and maritime pine bark and grape seed extract. An independent study on antioxidants has been conducted by Russian biochemists. As they announce their findings to the World Health

---

[160] **Majeed, Muhammed, Ph.D et al** *Curcuminoids – Antioxidant Phytonutrients,* Nutriscience Publishers, 121 Ethel Road West, Unit 6, Piscataway, NJ 08854 USA

Organisation, Revenol is expected to be listed as the world's No. 1 effective antioxidant.

Cascading Revenol (Neways International)
Neways has also released an exciting, further version of Revenol, named Cascading Revenol. Oxidation elements, or free radicals as they are sometimes known, are unpaired oxygen molecules which are hungry to scavenge additional oxygen, damage healthy cells and are especially dangerous for cancer sufferers. Antioxidants such as Vitamin C neutralise the damage caused by free radicals. The problem is, after having entered the body, most antioxidant molecular structures will grab one free radical and then change into an inert state, ceasing to be of further radical-scavenging value. The additional problem is that even when an antioxidant neutralises a free radical, the process creates an off-shoot free radical that is slightly different and less potent in variety, which in turn creates another, and so on. Typical antioxidants have no ability to address this free radical cascading effect.

However Cascading Revenol's technologically advanced formulation has been designed to regenerate these scavenging molecules so that they can neutralise multiple free radicals. So, instead of only one free radical being destroyed per antioxidant molecule, each molecule is able to change structure and repeat the process again and again. Thus the value of each individual antioxidant molecule increases exponentially. Cascading Revenol's unique action is devastating to the free radical onslaught that damages cancer sufferers and in my opinion is an essential component in any B17 Metabolic Therapy treatment.

Cassie-Tea (Neways International)
Cassie-Tea is a traditional health formula designed to help assist the body's efforts to eliminate toxins that accumulate in the body with age. Turkey rhubarb root supports liver and intestinal health, while sheep sorrel herb and burdock root help in the body's efforts to maintain the blood stream. Slippery Elm helps soothe

irritated mucus membranes and soothe and moisten the respiratory tract.

Neways' Cassie-Tea is the same as the famous Essiac. René Caisse, a Canadian nurse, treated thousands of cancer patients for sixty years using a herbal drink popular with the Ojibway Indians. In 1937 the Royal Cancer Commission of Canada conducted hearings concerning Essiac ('Caisse' backwards) and pronounced as its conclusion that the preparation had marked anti-cancer properties. Tom Mower, the president of Neways, obtained the formulation for Cassie-Tea from a source that used to mix the tea for Nurse Caisse. Cassie-Tea is an excellent nutritional supplement for those undergoing B17 Metabolic Therapy.

Hawaiian Noni Juice (Neways International)

The fruit juice of *Morinda citrifolia* contains a polysaccharide-rich substance with marked anti-tumour activity, according to recent studies into the famous fruit[161]. This research, performed at the University of Hawaii, has resulted in exciting new and scientifically reputable evidence for the potential benefits of Noni fruit juice in the treatment of cancer. Neways Authentic Hawaiian Noni features all the health-enhancing benefits of the noni plant as well as raspberry and blueberry extracts – both powerful antioxidants.

Purge / Feelin' Good (Neways International)

Researchers state that the majority of people, especially those with cancer, play host to one form of parasite or another. Parasites are life-forms that are uninvited lodgers in our bodies who do not pay rent. They can range from tiny amoebae detectable only with a microscope to tapeworms many feet in length.

We inadvertently pick up parasites through our day-to-day activities and especially through eating undercooked or contaminated food. Try an experiment and put some cat food out in

---

[161] **Hirazumi, A & Eiichi Furusawa** "An Immunomodulatory Polysaccharide-Rich Substance from the Fruit Juice of *Morinda citrifolia* (Noni) with Antitumour Activity", Dept of Pharmacology, John A Burns School of Medicine, Hawaii, HI 96822 USA

an isolated part of your yard for a few sunny days and then go back and examine it (don't let any pets interfere and keep away from grass and earth). You will invariably find it crawling with infestation.

Blood flukes can enter our systems through infected drinking water and take up residence in the bladder, intestines, liver, lungs, rectum and spleen, laying their eggs and breeding in humans for up to 20 years. Trichina worm larvae found in undercooked pork migrate from the intestines through the blood and lymphatic system, eventually lodging in muscles. Threadworm larvae enter skin from the soil and pass through the bloodstream to the lungs, sometimes causing pneumonia.

Eliminating parasites is effectively a three-phase program. Killing them, flushing them out and then supplementing our relieved bodies with healthy nutrients to maintain optimum health. Neways features this very effective three-phase program, employing their products Purge, Feelin' Good and Maximol Solutions respectively to execute the clean-up, leaving you bug-free and, most importantly, invigorated and strengthened to avoid re-infestation.

D-Toxarate (Neways International)
As we have already learned, every day we are exposed to harmful substances in our environment. The air we breathe, the food we eat, and even objects we touch are contaminated by substances that threaten our health in many ways we are only just beginning to understand. D-Toxarate is formulated with two important ingredients to help many of these substances pass through the body without harmful effects. Calcium d-glucarate, the first ingredient, can help eliminate some agents that potentially harm our cells. The second ingredient is ascorbic acid, or vitamin C, an antioxidant with another interesting property - it reduces blood-lead levels.

Calcium d-glucarate is a bioavailable salt of D-glucuronic acid. D-glucuronic acid is found naturally in fruits and vegetables, including oranges, spinach, apples, carrots, potatoes, and broccoli.[162] In the body, D-glucuronic acid breaks down into three components. The active component is D-glucaro-1,4-lactone, a substance important to the final stage of glucuronidation, one of the body's detoxification processes.

Vegetables and Fruits with High D-Glucaric Acid Content

Fruit/Vegetable	g/kg food
Grapefruit	3.60
Cactus (edible)	3.49
Macintosh Apple	3.45
Alfalfa Sprouts	3.45
Broccoli	3.40
Granny Smith Apple	3.36
Azuki bean Sprouts	2.78
Brussels Sprouts	2.67
Red Delicious Apple	2.26

During the glucuronidation process, environmental carcinogens such as polycyclic aromatic hydrocarbons, nitrosamines, aromatic amines, and fungal toxins enter the body and are glucuronidated. Glucuronidation increases the water-solubility of these carcinogens, thus reducing their carcinogenicity, and facilitating their expulsion from the body through the kidneys and bladder. Steroid hormones, which in excess may promote breast and prostate cancer, are also removed from the body through glucuronidation.

Calcium d-glucarate has also been shown to encourage the differentiation of rat mammary cells.[163] Healthy cells differentiate and perform special functions depending upon their type. Cancer cells do not differentiate.

---

[162] **Dwivedi C, Heck WJ, Downie AA, Larroya S, Webb TE** "Effect of calcium glucarate on beta-glucuronidase activity and glucarate content of certain vegetables and fruits." *Biochem Med Metab Biol* 1990 Apr;43(2):83-92.
[163] **Abou-Issa H, Moeschberger M, Ei-Masry W, Tejwani S, Curley RW, Webb TE** "Relative Efficacy of Glucarate on the Initiation and Promotion Phases of Rat Mammary Carcinogenesis." *Anticancer Research.* 1995;15:805-810.

In addition to its cancer preventative properties, calcium d-glucarate is a source of calcium, a nutrient essential for the healthy functioning of neurons, muscles, and bones.

Vitamin C has been included in the formula to protect against lead—another harmful substance. It is well known that lead toxicity is dangerous, especially to children. Even low levels of lead can have neuropsychological effects, reduce stature, and increase incidence of dental caries.[164] Although exposure to lead has been reduced significantly by removing it from common household items, exposure to lead still occurs from previously contaminated paint and soil (see Vitamin C in this section).

Supplementation with D-Toxarate can be beneficial to anyone concerned by environmental pollution. It may be particularly beneficial taken in conjunction with an antioxidant formula such as Cascading Revenol. Calcium d-glucarate benefits persons exposed to environmental carcinogens such as cigarette smoke and other industrial pollutants, persons with low intake of D-glucuronic acid from natural substances (less than 5 fruits and vegetables containing high levels of D-glucuronic acid per day), or persons with high beta-glucuronidase activity. Vitamin C supplementation benefits anyone concerned with exposure to lead.

VitaCell - Resveratrol, Maitake, Lycopene combination (Neways International)

The human body is a miraculous system of organs, with several different mechanisms for removing harmful substances from the body, repairing damaged cells or accidental mutations, replacing older cells with new cells, and removing ill or dead cells from the body. Three novel substances have recently gained attention in the scientific community for their potential anti-cancer activity: resveratrol, maitake mushroom, and lycopene. Together, these products act as antioxidants, detoxify through the enzymatic pathway, protect hormone receptors, encourage cells to go through

---

[164] **Matte TD** "Reducing Blood Lead Levels." *JAMA*. 1999;281:2340-2342.

natural differentiation and apoptosis processes, and support the immune system's efforts to police the entire system.

Resveratrol is a phytoalexin, the component of plants that protects them from fungal infections. It is found abundantly in *Polygonum cuspidatum* root (a Chinese medicinal plant) and is also a component of other fruits and vegetables, most notably grapes. The roots of *Polygonum cuspidatum* have been used traditionally in Asian medicine for conditions such as rheumatism, cough, burn, or ulcer.[165] Additionally, resveratrol has been brought to the spotlight as one of the main ingredients which scientists have studied in relation to the cardiovascular benefits of alcohol, particularly red wine. Recently, resveratrol has been studied as a possible chemopreventive agent. Although studies suggest multiple mechanisms of action, there is general agreement that resveratrol stops initiation, promotion, and progression of cancer. Most of the studies to date have been performed *in vitro* using doses of resveratrol that could be achieved through a diet high in grapes or grape products.

Maitake mushroom (*Grifola frondosa*) has been eaten as food in Japan for hundreds of years, some people eating up to several hundred grams per day.[166] It contains a polysaccharide known as beta-glucan with immunostimulatory effects. Many mushrooms contain types of beta-glucans; however Maitake contains the most effective beta-glucan and is orally available.[167] A combination of Maitake beta-glucan and Vitamin C induced greater than 90% cell death in androgen-independent prostatic cancer PC-3 cells at clinically achievable concentrations.[168] Studies in mice show that, depending on the type of tumour, maitake inhibits tumor growth

---

[165] **Tang W, Eisenbrand G** "Chinese Drugs of Plant Origin: Chemistry, Pharmacology, and Use in Traditional and Modern Medicine." London: Springer-Verlag, 1992, 787-789.

[166] **Kidd PM** "The Use of Mushroom Glucans and Proteoglycans in Cancer Treatment." *Altern Med Rev* 2000 Feb;5(1):4-27.

[167] **Nanba H** "Activity of Maitake D-fraction to Inhibit Carcinogenesis and Metastasis." *Ann N Y Acad Sci* 1995 Sep;768:243-245.

[168] **Fullerton SA, Samadi AA, Tortorelis DG, et al** "Induction of Apoptosis in Human Prostatic Cancer Cells with Beta-Glucan (Maitake Mushroom Polysaccharide." *Molecular Urology* 2000 Nov;4(1):7-13.

from 27% to 75%.[169] Maitake's effects on tumor growth appear to be linked to the immune system. Maitake stimulates macrophages and T cells,[170] which are important elements in the body's immune system. Macrophages engulf unhealthy cells and remove them from the body.

Lycopene is a member of the carotene family. It is the red pigment found in fruits such as tomatoes and tomato products, apricots, pink grapefruit, guava, watermelon, and papaya. Over 85% of consumed lycopene is found in processed tomato products.[171] Many epidemiological studies have examined the relationship between the intake of tomatoes, tomato-based products, or lycopene and incidence of various cancers. A recent review of 72 such studies found that 57 studies reported that higher tomato intake or blood lycopene level decreased risk of cancer. For 35 studies, this relationship was statistically significant. No studies showed an increased risk of cancer due to tomato intake or blood lycopene level. The evidence was strongest for prostate, lung, and stomach cancer.[172]

Over time, as the body is bombarded with carcinogens and goes through the normal cycles of cell life and death, the likelihood of developing abnormal cells increases. Thus, during mid-life and beyond, it is necessary to increase intake of substances that prevent the promotion and progression of abnormal cell growth. VitaCell can benefit anyone concerned that their exposure to carcinogens has been high or who has low intake of these substances in their normal diet. The benefits of Maitake mushroom may be improved by concurrent Vitamin C supplementation.

---

[169] **Hishida I, Nanba H, Kuroda H** "Antitumor Activity Exhibited by Orally Administered Extract from Fruit Body of *Grifola frondosa* (Maitake)." *Chem Pharm Bull* 1988;36(5):1819-1827.

[170] **Nanba H, Keiko K.** "Effect of Maitake D-Fraction on Cancer Prevention." *Ann N Y Acad Sci* 1997 Dec;833:204-207.

[171] **Gerster H** "The Potential Role of Lycopene for Human Health." *Journal of the American College of Nutrition* 1997;16(2):109-126.

[172] **Giovannucci E** "Tomatoes, Tomato-Based Products, Lycopene, and Cancer: review of the Epidemiologic Literature." *Journal of the National Cancer Institute* 1999 Feb;91(4):317-331.

Dimethyl sulfoxide (DMSO)

DMSO is a by-product of the wood and paper industry and has gained prominence in recent times as a highly effective agent in the treatment of herpes, cancer and other diseases. DMSO is a unique solvent that penetrates the blood/brain barrier and is used with B17 intravenously to deliver the principal treatment deep into the body without changing the latter's chemical structure. DMSO is renowned for its ability to penetrate the body's tissue rapidly and completely. Credence has a special report on DMSO which can be obtained free by e-mailing us your request at dmso@credence.org.

Vitamin C (Ascorbic acid)

Dr Linus Pauling, often known as the 'Father of Vitamin C' and twice awarded the Nobel Prize for his work in medicine, declared that large intakes of up to 10g of the vitamin each day aids anti-cancer activity within the body. Pauling was largely derided for making these declarations, but today, large doses of Vitamin C are used by many practitioners for cancer patients in nutritional therapy, who believe Pauling was right and that the popular nutrient is indispensable to the body in its fight to regain health from cancer.

Several studies have suggested that Vitamin C may reduce levels of lead in the blood. Epidemiological studies have shown that people with elevated blood serum levels of Vitamin C had lower levels of blood toxicity. An examination of the data from the Third National Health and Nutrition Examination Survey, enrolling 4,213 youths aged 6 to 16 years and 15,365 adults 17 years and older from 1988 to 1994, found a correlation between low serum ascorbic acid levels and elevated blood lead levels. The authors conclude that high ascorbic acid intake may reduce blood lead levels.[173]

An analysis of the Normative Aging Study, which enrolled 747 men aged 49 to 93 years from 1991 to 1995, found that lower

---

[173] **Simon JA, Hudes ES** "Relationship of Ascorbic Acid to Blood Lead Levels." *JAMA.* 1999;281:2289-2293.

dietary intake of Vitamin C may increase lead levels in the blood.[174] A study of 349 African American women enrolled in the project Nutrition, Other Factors, and the Outcome of Pregnancy found that vitamin-mineral supplementation resulted in increased serum levels of ascorbic acid and decreased serum levels of lead. The authors concluded that maternal use of a vitamin supplement with ascorbic acid and vitamin E might offer protection from lead contamination of the foetus during pregnancy.[175]

Because smoking lowers levels of ascorbic acid in the body, researchers theorised that Vitamin C supplementation may effect blood lead levels in smokers. A clinical study was performed on 75 adult men 20 to 30 years of age who smoked at least one pack of cigarettes per day, but had no clinical signs of ascorbic acid deficiency or lead toxicity. Subjects were randomly assigned to daily supplementation with placebo, 200 mg of ascorbic acid, or 1000 mg of ascorbic acid. After one week of supplementation, there was an 81% decrease in blood-lead levels in the group taking 1000 mg of ascorbic acid daily.[176]

Dosage recommended by Linus Pauling is up to 10g/day. High levels of Vitamin C however can cause diarrhoea and may be contra-indicated with certain chemotherapy treatments. Vitamin C is especially useful when combined in moderate amounts with Calcium d-glucarate, as formulated in the Neways product D-Toxarate (see D-Toxarate in this section).

Implementing Changes - Convert Your Bathroom Pack
As many of the harmful ingredients we examined earlier can be found in the average bathroom, clear these out in one fell swoop.

---

[174] **Cheng Y, Willett WC, Schwartz J, Sparrow D, Weiss S, Hu H** "Relation of nutrition to bone lead and blood lead levels in middle-aged to elderly men. The Normative Aging Study." *Am J Epidemiol* 1998 Jun 15;147(12):1162-1174.

[175] **West WL, Knight EM, Edwards CH, et al.** "Maternal low level lead and pregnancy outcomes." *J Nutr.* 1994 Jun;124(6 Suppl):981S-986S.

[176] **Dawson EB, Evans DR, Harris WA, Teter MC, McGanity WJ** "The effect of ascorbic acid supplementation on the blood lead levels of smokers." *J Am Coll Nutr.* 1999 Apr;18(2):166-170.

At the moment, many of us are brushing our teeth with rat poison, washing our hair out with cheap engine degreasants, putting liquid paraffin on our babies in the form of baby oil, firing aluminium into our lymph nodes under our arms and using constituents of brake fluid and antifreeze in our make-up and personal care formulae.

Neways' Convert Your Bathroom pack contains shampoo, conditioner, bath gel, shaving gel, deodorant, toothpaste and mouthwash that are not only free from damaging ingredients, but are of the highest quality. Whether you are undergoing nutritional therapy for cancer or are simply interested in cancer prevention, the cumulative toxic onslaught your body receives at the hands of harmful consumer products has to stop.

Implementing Changes – Importance of Diet

Changes in diet are essential to avoid contracting a deficiency disease. As we have seen, the main culprit is the good old Western diet, heavy in meats, sugars, fats and chemicals. Removal of almost all meats, as well as toxic foodstuffs such as additives, caffeine, refined sugars and chocolate represents a major start. Weight loss and a return of energy are almost immediate, and with these benefits comes a regular method of detoxifying the body as part of your future lifestyle. Once again, fruit only before noon, followed by a properly combined diet, low in meats (if you need to eat them) and rich in unrefined and, where possible, uncooked plant dietary. The body takes in its amino acids ideally from high quality vegetation, fruits and nuts. From these aminos we then construct our human proteins accordingly.

The Nutrition Police are not going to cuff you and take you off to jail if you slip up. I always advise that folks try this new eating lifestyle for a minimum of four weeks to test it out and become familiar with the concepts of Natural Hygiene, as it is known.

Rapid detoxification can be achieved simply by eating more fruit in the morning between when you awaken and noon. Fruits such as pineapple, grapes (eat the seeds!), plums and oranges are among many that are ideal for this purpose and contain a vast array of nutrients, whose effectiveness and modality are only now beginning to be properly understood. If you are used to bulk in the mornings with the traditional breakfasts, eat more fruit and then wait for your raised blood sugars to remove your feelings of hunger. For concrete advice on these highly effective dietary regimens, and what to do if you are diabetic, we recommend Harvey and Marilyn Diamond's *Fit For Life* series of books (see bibliography).

Exercise in Moderation

Research shows that those with a sedentary lifestyle are more prone to cancer and heart problems. A moderate exercise program will assist in cleansing the body and getting all the pieces of the body toned and in proper working order. Simply MOVE! Walking, a non-threatening hour in the gym twice or three times a week or cycling are ideal and immensely enjoyable once you get on the pro-active program. If you sit still all day long, you might as well not breathe! Life is about healthy action. Celebrate your life by looking, moving and feeling the way your body was designed to be.

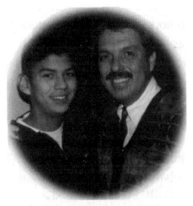

Charlie Molina and Dr Francisco Contreras of the Oasis Clinic. Charlie was diagnosed with Hodgkins Disease in 1991. Today he is a cancer-free 17 year-old boy.

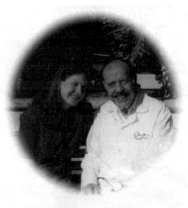

Sarah Sackett and Dr. Ernesto Contreras, Sr.

"I've been free of cancer since 1991. I love God and I love my doctor!"

Sarah

Sarah Sackett was another who found life at Oasis. Sarah is pictured here with one of the world's original pioneers of Metabolic Therapy, Dr Ernesto Contreras.

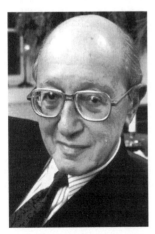

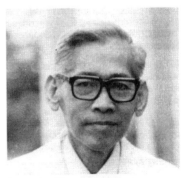

Dr Manuel Navarro
Over 25 years of experience with amygdalin and detecting early cancers with the HCG test

Dr Samuel Epstein is a tireless crusader to alert the public of the dangers of environmental contaminants. His book, *The Politics of Cancer (Revisited)* gives startling information on industry's widespread abuses

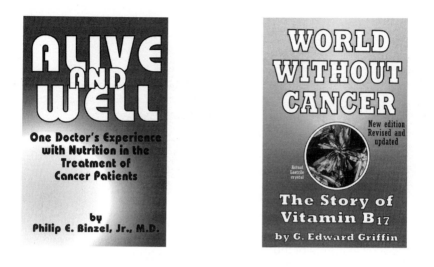

Dr Philip Binzel's *Alive & Well* and Edward Griffin's *World Without Cancer* are recommended for an in-depth analysis of the nutritional therapy story. Griffin reports also John Richardson's work and touches on aspects of Metabolic Therapy nutrition more roundly expounded in June de Spain's *Little Cyanide Cookbook* and Harvey and Marilyn Diamond's *Fit For Life* (these titles are available through Credence Publications at www.credence.org)

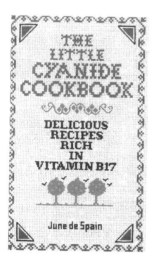

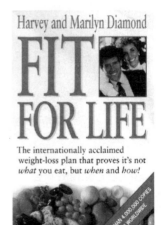

Why Are The Nations Dying?

Degenerative diseases are taking hold of industrialised nations like never before. The following excerpted US Senate document warned of the health holocaust to come.

Senate Document No. 264, 1936.

74th Congress, 2nd Session

"Our physical well-being is more directly dependent upon minerals we take into our systems than upon calories or vitamins, or upon precise proportions of starch, protein or carbohydrates we consume... Do you know that most of us today are suffering from certain dangerous diet deficiencies which cannot be remedied until depleted soils from which our food comes are brought into proper mineral balance?

The alarming fact is that foods (fruits, vegetables and grains), now being raised on millions of acres of land that no longer contain enough of certain minerals, are starving us - no matter how much of them we eat. No man of today can eat enough fruits and vegetables to supply his system with the minerals he requires for perfect health because his stomach isn't big enough to hold them.

The truth is, our foods vary enormously in value, and some of them aren't worth eating as food... Our physical well-being is more directly dependent upon the minerals we take into our systems than upon calories or vitamins or upon the precise proportions of starch, protein or carbohydrates we consume.

This talk about minerals is novel and quite startling. In fact, a realization of the importance of minerals in food is so new that the text books on nutritional dietetics contain very little about it. Nevertheless, it is something that concerns all of us, and the further we delve into it the more startling it becomes.

You'd think, wouldn't you, that a carrot is a carrot - that one is about as good as another as far as nourishment is concerned? But it isn't; one carrot may look and taste like another and yet be lacking in the particular mineral element which our system requires and which carrots are supposed to contain.

Laboratory test prove that the fruits, the vegetables, the grains, the eggs, and even the milk and the meats of today are not what they were a few generations ago (which doubtless explains why our forefathers thrived on a selection of foods that would starve us!)

No man today can eat enough fruits and vegetables to supply his stomach with the mineral salts he requires for perfect health, because his stomach isn't big enough to hold them! And we are turning into big stomachs.

No longer does a balanced and fully nourishing diet consist merely of so many calories or certain vitamins or fixed proportion of starches, proteins and carbohydrates. We know that our diets must contain in addition something like a score of minerals salts.

It is bad news to learn from our leading authorities that 99% of the American people are deficient in these minerals [this was in 1936!], **and that a marked deficiency in any one of the more important minerals actually results in disease. Any upset of the balance, any considerable lack or one or another element, however microscopic the body requirement may be, and we sicken, suffer, shorten our lives.**

We know that vitamins are complex chemical substances which are indispensable to nutrition, and that each of them is of importance for normal function of some special structure in the body. Disorder and disease result from any vitamin deficiency. **It is not commonly realized, however, that vitamins control the body's appropriation of minerals, and in the absence of minerals they have no function to perform. Lacking vitamins, the system can make some use of minerals, but lacking minerals, vitamins are useless. Certainly our physical well-being is more directly dependent upon the minerals we take into our systems than upon calories of vitamins or upon the precise proportions of starch, protein of carbohydrates we consume.**

This discovery is one of the latest and most important contributions of science to the problem of human health."

Scurvy – A Parable of Entrenched Error

According to naval records, over one million British sailors died of scurvy between 1600 and 1800. Yet for hundreds of years the cure for this gum-rotting and organ-destroying disease had already been part of the official record.

In the winter of 1535, French explorer Jacques Cartier found himself stranded when his ship became trapped in the ice in a tributary of the St Lawrence River. Soon his crew began dying of scurvy. Out of an original ship's complement of a hundred and ten men, twenty-five had already perished of the disease and many others were so sick they were not expected to recover.

Believing that the condition was caused by bad vapours or some malignant cause to do with the 'sea airs', Cartier was astonished when help came from an unexpected direction. Some friendly local Indians showed Cartier how to boil pine needles and bark from the white pine, later found to be rich in Vitamin C[177]. His sailors swiftly recovered after drinking the beverage. Upon his return, Cartier enthusiastically reported this miraculous cure to medical authorities. The latter merely laughed at his "witchdoctors' curses of ignorant savages" and did nothing about the information they were given, except to log it into their records.

Scurvy had traditionally been a fatal scourge to seafarers. Between 1497 and 1499, veteran Portuguese explorer Vasco da Gama lost over a hundred men to the disease on one voyage alone, once again believing as medicine did at the time, that some lurking 'vapour' in the holds of ships or contagion was the cause. Sir Richard Hawkins, the famous British Elizabethan admiral, faced scurvy among his crew on a lengthy voyage to Brazil and discovered that eating oranges and lemons cured the condition immediately. However, despite reporting this phenomenon to the British Admiralty and to any physicians who would listen, this valuable knowledge perished along with Hawkins.

Deaths from scurvy became so numerous that by the eighteenth century more British sailors were dying from ascorbic acid deficiency than

---

[177] Interestingly, the main ingredients in the pine needles and bark offered to Cartier's sailors are contained in the powerful antioxidant product, Revenol, manufactured and distributed by Neways.

were being killed in combat. Between 1740 and 1744, British admiral George A Anson set sail to circumnavigate the globe in his flagship *Centurion.* Originally starting with six ships and almost 2,000 healthy men, *Centurion* was the only ship that eventually returned. Anson reported that scurvy alone had killed over 1,000 of his men.

Such was the turmoil and embarrassment this event caused in British Admiralty circles that a naval surgeon, John Lind, became determined to find the cure for the dreaded disease. On 20th May 1747, Lind commenced an experiment which dramatically demonstrated that fresh greens and plenty of fruits eaten by scurvy sufferers produced stunning recoveries. Later experiments clearly showed that those who ate a balanced diet, fortified with these vegetable and fruit elements, did not contract scurvy.

Yet what was the reaction of the establishment? The British Admiralty and numerous other physicians, who had individually been attempting to solve the same problem and thus earn grants and fame, barely gave Lind's findings any credence. It took 48 more years and thousands of further scurvy deaths before his advice finally became official Navy quartermaster policy. Ironically, after implementing this simple measure, the British, who became known as 'limeys' because of their new nutrition procedure, soon gained strategic ascendancy on the world's seas, building the greatest empire the world has ever seen. After 1800, British sailors never contracted scurvy. The naval might of Britain's enemies however continued to be decimated by it. Author Edward Griffin remarks: *"It is no exaggeration to say that the greatness of the British Empire in large measure was the direct result of overcoming scientific prejudice against vitamin therapy[178]."*

One would have thought that the scurvy matter ended there. One would be wrong. As the obsession with virus and microbe hunting began to grip developing medicine during the late nineteenth century, it was easier to find a bacterium than to isolate the elusive vitamin. Scientists became distracted. Suddenly a simple nutritional deficiency no longer seemed a plausible, complete answer to scurvy. It had to be something more complicated. As science proceeded, so came the problems. The new pasteurisation techniques for milk unwittingly destroyed its ascorbic acid content, leading to hundreds of fresh scurvy cases among children each year.

---

[178] Griffin, G Edward, ibid. p.54

174

Professor CP Stewart of Edinburgh University remarks: *"One factor which undoubtedly held up the development of the concept of deficiency diseases was the discovery of bacteria in the nineteenth century and the consequent preoccupation of scientists and doctors with positive infective agents in disease. So strong was the impetus provided by bacteriology that many diseases which we now know to be due to nutritional or endocrine deficiencies were, as late as 1910, thought to be "toxemias"; in default of any evidence of an active infecting micro-organism, they were ascribed to the remote effects of imaginary toxins elaborated by bacteria[179]."*

With medicine's attention taken from Lind's earlier findings with fruit and vegetables, scurvy began to rear its ugly head once more as emphasis on the importance of diet lapsed. During World War 1, Russian soldiers suffered miserably from scurvy, their appalling conditions primarily being blamed as the cause. Fortunately, the search for Vitamin C was not to be permanently derailed by grant-hungry microbe hunters and by the 1930s, purified Vitamin C had been successfully isolated and scurvy was officially declared vanquished.

From the time the cure had become known in Europe, all it had taken to conquer scurvy was 450 years, millions of deaths, and finally the belief in a simple diet of fruit.

---

[179] **Stewart, CP** and D Guthrie, *Lind's Treatise on Scurvy,* Edinburgh University Press, 1953 pp. 408-409

Swimming Against the Tide
A report by Tina Cooke

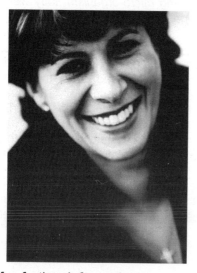

In January 1999 I was diagnosed with an aggressive form of breast cancer. I underwent three major surgeries and was supposed to follow through the course of six chemotherapies, radiation and a stem cell transplant. Vulnerable as you are when diagnosed and given an extremely poor prognosis, I agreed to any form of treatment my surgeons and oncologists saw fit. In hindsight, I realise that I must have taken leave of my senses. Never once did I question them, or ask them for further information or papers on the chemotherapy substances they would be using, such as Tamoxifen[180]. Like so many others, I have children, am 42 years old, and have a job. To be told that your odds of living are 30 percent in the first five years is pretty grim. So in the end, because I wanted to survive, the doctors had my full co-operation to do whatever they wanted.

I got through the surgeries, amputee that I am, but I could live with that. But I managed just three of the six chemotherapies. The first one was a doddle. I had no problem with it, and thought that if that was all there was to it, well I can handle it! I read and read orthodox books.

The second chemo took its toll. I began to flare up with fungi growing over my body. My hair began rapidly to fall out – it was so

---

[180] Tamoxifen......

heartbreaking, but a small price to pay, or so I thought. Rashes appeared all over my body. The nausea and tiredness took their toll. By the third chemo, I was unrecognisable, visually and mentally. I was despondent, lost my will, was losing weight, and physically finding it difficult to cope. The worst pain was not being able to live a normal life with my children. So here I was spending the last years of my life in misery, with my kids accepting that their mother was no longer theirs as they knew her.

By a twist of good luck and with a prayer to God, I was fortunate enough to bump into two old school friends whose father, Teddy Goldsmith, was the owner and publisher of the *Ecologist* magazine[181]. I had been aware of this publication since my school days and knew that it dealt with matters of the environment. But like most people who live in a cocooned existence, magazines like his didn't really mean much to me. I had never read anything to do with degenerative diseases, let alone the potential of the harm we as humans were doing to ourselves by abusing the environment. But Teddy had vision. He didn't have any aspirations to be a politician or make money out of informing people of the impending hazards associated with our world. He just wanted people to understand that we should behave more responsibly towards our environment and try and look after ourselves and our children for the future. To me this man has been my saviour.

Teddy gave me a copy of one of his issues, *Cancer - Are the Experts Lying?*[182] I looked at the copy for several days and finally found the energy and the will to read it. I was horrified. This man was able to explain to me that cancer didn't need to be so debilitating. That cancer could be controlled, but not the orthodox way as we all knew it. But how?

It was all there. Factual information about how the pharmaceutical industry worked, about alternative treatments

---

[181] The Ecologist magazine regularly champions the cause of exposing the effects of environmental carcinogens and is an excellent resource for those wishing to learn more. Visit their site at www.theecologist.com.

[182] *The Ecologist*, Vol.28, No. 2, March/April 1998 Fax +44(0)1258 473476, e-mail ecologist@gn.apc.org

available in other countries, statistics showing that thousands and thousands of people were being cured by natural methods and what cancer meant to the pharmaceutical industry.

I remembered a conversation I had with my oncologist. He had said: *"If you were my daughter, although the stem cell treatment is experimental, I would suggest you have it in the light of your poor prognosis. It will cost you in the region of £25,000 but I believe you will be able to recoup some of this through your insurance company."*

It suddenly dawned on me. Cancer really was a business. Was it possible that the experts knew what they were doing to us? I believe they do. How many times do you see headlines breaking news like... *"Cancer Breakthrough! New drug shows promise of curing cancer - the magic bullet."* Two days later, there will be further front-page news on how successful the experiments were on mice. Two days later... *"Sorry, unfortunately this treatment will not be available for at least ten years, and anyway we don't know if it will have the same success results on humans as it does with mice."* Watch the share price of the drug company concerned!

In the end I made the decision to travel to Mexico to be treated with B17 Metabolic Therapy at Stella Maris, one of the 20 or so hugely popular Tijuana cancer clinics specialising in alternative cancer therapies. The treatments I received included the replacement of mercury amalgam tooth fillings, intravenous drips of laetrile, enzymes and antioxidants, a complete change of diet, including organic fruits and vegetables. I also received other complementary therapies, including DMSO (dimethylsulfoxide), Vitamin C, lymphatic massage and daily supplements individually tailored for each patient. Within one week, the change was evident to all, including a *Daily Mail* journalist who had flown to Mexico to record my progress for a forthcoming article in her paper's Sunday magazine, *"You"*. My mouth ulcer had cleared up, my hair was looking more lustrous and I was full of energy for the first time in months.

I returned to England a new woman. My cancer was not yet cured, but controlled. After months of questions, investigation, checking and re-checking, I decided to form the Cancer Alternative Information Bureau (CAIB). It is not a charity but merely an information bureau where I can share what I have found with anyone who wishes to know. My search has led me to identify some brilliant doctors, who had, like me, also become disillusioned with the orthodox approach to cancer, who even today work tirelessly with alternative therapies, achieving good results in this field. Cancer cannot always be cured but it certainly can be controlled.

With breast cancer we now find that the death rate is escalating out of control, especially in England. HRH The Prince of Wales announced in England recently that he would become patron of *Breakthrough*, a research organisation dedicated to finding the cause of cures for breast cancer. Many celebrities are supportive of this organisation, but most have not yet had the courage to come forward and help us make a stand against the intransigence of the cancer industry.

I believe the time has come for the blinkers to come off and for the truth about ALL cancer treatments to emerge. The age-old cliché still holds true – THE PEOPLE HAVE THE RIGHT TO KNOW. My hope is that you will find our organisation of great use in helping you to become educated about this subject through our information pack and books like the one you are currently reading. There is great hope here! Help us spread the word. Help us spread the hope of life.

Kind regards
Tina Cooke

IF I CAN DO IT, SO CAN YOU!

By Hilary Englefield

I was shattered when I was told I had cancer. The doctor said I had to have a radical mastectomy on the right breast and a partial mastectomy on the left breast. This surgical procedure would then probably be followed by chemotherapy, radiotherapy, or both, and removal of the lymph nodes if this was deemed necessary. I had previously requested a blood test, but was told that there was no specific blood test available.

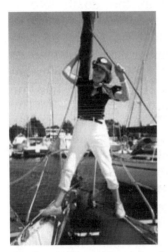

It was obvious from the Internet that people in America treat many different types of cancer with a non-carcinogenic, organic diet and vitamins and minerals, plus other natural plant extracts, and I contacted some of the organisations promoting these therapies. They were wonderfully supportive. Tina Cooke, who had been to Mexico for treatment, also gave me immediate help and advice about her regimen. I remembered a book called *Killing Cancer*, by Jason Winters, in which he described searching all over the world for a cure, and how he found the ingredients for a herbal tea which is known to kill cancer cells.

I sought a second opinion, which proved to be very negative, during which the oncologist repeated that there was no specific blood test available that would show whether the cancer cells were proliferating. This, I later discovered, was not correct, as a blood test had been developed in 1998 in the USA, and was available in England through London laboratories.

I then decided to seek a third opinion from another doctor. I had known her for many years, and felt I could rely on her implicitly. She confirmed that I had Paget's disease of the nipple, which could produce multiple tumours overnight and spread rapidly (in fact, I had suffered from this disease already for four months, since June, when I was referred to the cancer clinic). Together we designed a program of treatment including Vitamins A, C, E, all the B's, magnesium, betaine, folic acid, linseed oil capsules and other items. One of the main therapies we used was intravenous amygdalin (vitamin B17), which I obtained from America and gave to the doctor, who administered it on alternate days. I attended the hospital each day as an out-patient.

I started my treatment program in mid-November 1998, and within a fortnight, I felt 20 years younger. For the previous 18 years I had also suffered from ME (chronic fatigue). The cancer treatment and nutritional supplementation I received, I believe to this day, was responsible for clearing 95% of my chronic fatigue symptoms. In February 1999 my blood test results were normal; the cancer had regressed and was not now apparent. My intravenous injections were gradually reduced, one by one, and I have now ceased my hospital treatment. My oral supplements, which I take at home, include vitamins and minerals, plus other natural plant extracts. I also take Jason Winter's tea, and Essiac, a similar tea based on a formula an ex-nurse discovered in Canada.

I now anticipate being alive to see my grandchildren grow up and would advise anyone in a similar position to seek a second or even third opinion, until they are satisfied that the information they are given is correct. One book in particular I recommend for solid advice on cancer treatment alternatives is Phillip Day's *Cancer: Why We're Still Dying to Know the Truth.* I was convinced that there had to be an alternative to surgery and chemotherapy. I hope my testimony gives people hope, and the chance to say, "If she can do it, why can't 1?"

Hilary Englefield is founder of the Hope Trust (Chichester), UK registered charity # 1058637. Hilary's organisation is dedicated to promoting natural, effective treatments for diseases.

American Cancer Society Indicted

CHICAGO, 25th Oct 1999 /PRNewswire/ - The following was released today by the Cancer Prevention Coalition:

An article, "American Cancer Society: The World's Wealthiest 'Non-Profit' Institution," by Dr Samuel Epstein, just published in the *International Journal of Health Services*, the leading international public health and policy journal, charges that the American Cancer Society (ACS) *"is fixated on damage control ... diagnosis and treatment ... and basic molecular biology, with indifference or even hostility to cancer prevention."* ACS also trivializes the escalating incidence of cancer which has reached epidemic proportions and makes grossly misleading claims on dramatic progress in the treatment and cure of cancer. This myopic mindset and derelict policy is compounded by interlocking conflicts of interests with the cancer drug, agrichemical, and other industries. The following is illustrative:

- ♦ Since 1982, the ACS has adopted a highly restrictive policy insisting on unequivocal human evidence on carcinogenicity before taking any position on cancer risks. Accordingly, the ACS has actively campaigned against the 1958 Delaney law banning the deliberate addition to food of any amount of chemical additive shown to induce cancer, even in well-validated federal animal tests.
- ♦ In a joint 1992 statement with the Chlorine Institute, the ACS supported the continued use of organochlorine pesticides in spite of their recognized environmental persistence and carcinogenicity.
- ♦ In 1993, just before PBS *Frontline* aired the special entitled "In Our Children's Food," the ACS sent a memorandum in support of the pesticide industry to some 48 regional divisions which pre-emptively trivialized pesticides as a cause of childhood cancer and reassured

182

the public that residues of carcinogenic pesticide in food are safe, even for babies.

♦ In *Cancer Facts & Figures*, the ACS annual publication designed to provide the public with "basic facts" on cancer, there is little or no mention of prevention. Examples include no mention of: dusting the genital area with talc as a known cause of ovarian cancer; parental exposure to occupational carcinogens, domestic use of pesticides, or frequent consumption of nitrite colored hot dogs (resultingly contaminated with carcinogenic nitrosamines) as major causes of childhood cancer; and prolonged use of oral contraceptives or hormonal replacement therapy as major causes of breast cancer. Facts & Figures, 1997, also misrepresented that *"since women may not be able to alter their personal risk factors, the best opportunity for reducing mortality is early detection."* This statement ignores overwhelming evidence on a wide range of ways by which women of all ages can reduce their risks of breast cancer, including regular use of the cheap non-prescription and safe drug aspirin.

♦ The ACS, together with the National Cancer Institute, has strongly promoted the use of Tamoxifen, the world's top-selling cancer drug, ($400 million annually) manufactured by Zeneca, for allegedly preventing breast cancer in healthy women, evidence for which is highly arguable at best. More seriously, ACS has trivialized the dangerous and sometimes lethal complications of Tamoxifen including blood clots, lung embolism, and aggressive uterine cancer, and fails to warn that the drug is a highly potent liver carcinogen.

Conflicts of interest are further reflected in the ACS Foundation Board of Trustees, which includes corporate executives from the pharmaceutical, cancer drug, investment, and media industries. They include David R. Bethume, president of Lederle Laboratories, Gordon Binder, CEO of Amgen (a leading biotech cancer drug company), and Sumner M. Redstone, chairman of the Board of Viacom, Inc.

Other concerns relate to the "non-profit status" of the ACS whose annual budget is some $500 million. Most funds raised go to pay high overhead, salaries, fringe benefits, and travel expenses of national executives in Atlanta, CEO's who earn six-figure salaries in several states, and hundreds of other employees working in some 3,000 regional offices. Less than 16% of all monies raised are spent on direct patient services; salaries and overhead for most ACS affiliates exceed 50%, although most direct community services are handled by unpaid volunteers. While ACS cash assets and reserves approach $1 billion, it continues to plead poverty and lament the lack of funds for cancer research. Not surprisingly, the Chronicle of Philanthropy, the leading U.S. charity watchdog, has concluded that the ACS is "more interested in accumulating wealth than saving lives." It should further be noted that the ACS uses 10 employees and spends $1 million a year on direct lobbying, and is the only known charity that makes contributions to political parties.

Based on these considerations the International Journal of Heath Services article urged that, in the absence of drastic reforms, contributions to the ACS should be diverted to public interest and environmental groups directly involved in cancer prevention. This is the only message that this "charity" can no longer ignore.

Testimonies

Jason Vale recovered from three bouts of 'terminal' cancer. Today he arm-wrestles nationally, is an active B17 campaigner, and hosts an Internet journal, recording day-to-day updates of the cancer sufferers with whom he comes into contact.

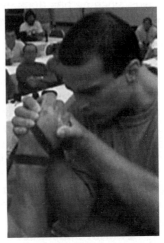

"I've been writing this journal and my name is Jason Vale, I've also had a 100% death-rate diagnosis and am perfectly fine now. I didn't have access to apricot seeds or vitamin B17 back then. I just went to the store and bought cases of peaches and broke open the pits and ate the seeds out. Supposedly if you're older it helps to have the B17 also because your body needs more help in the fight than with a younger person."

3rd November 1997

I spoke with **Tom Stratton, (RR1 Box 90 E, Constableville, NY 13325)** Tom had a large mole on his right back. He started only the seeds and in a few days he reported the outside of the spot drying up. In a couple of weeks it was smaller and the middle looked funny. I just spoke to Tom and he said the middle of the patch is back to normal skin.

Today I had a message that the FDA was at my house. I called Ken Kolas who has been raided by the FDA since he was 14 (his father won back all the property that they took after a long court battle) he said that they were just on a fact-finding mission. I'm pretty excited.

10th November 1997

Frank Jursits reports today that all tumors are now gone on right side of lung and a large nodule is still left on the left side. He has been taking the B17 and the seeds for two months. He's having a hard time. He started bleeding. Frank has already had one leg amputated due to cancer and has gone through the worst chemo and radiation. He was left terminal.

Charles Weiler had skin tumors (not cancerous) and they have all fallen off after 2 months of seeds and B17. **Charles Weiler, 20 Evergreen Lane. Hadean Field NJ 08033.**

My Father (**Joseph Vale**) has reported that he no longer has back pains since he has been eating the seeds for the last 3 months. Had this pain for years but isn't sure why. It's gone now.

11th November 1997

Toby Cederbaum called today and reported that the pain from the tumors in her breast is 75% gone. She never had them biopsied to see if they were definitely cancerous, but her mother and father died from cancer. They have all shrunk down more than half. She's only taking the seeds and not the vitamin. Her phone # is **(973)325 2117.** (Update on **Toby Cedarbaum** 3/10/98 spoke to her. She says that she stopped eating the seeds for a while after the tumors went away. She started eating bad and the pain came back in her breasts full force. She ate the seeds again and the pain went away immediately that day. She called crying almost and saying a sweet thank you).

21st November 1997

Today I received a call from **Jerry Butler, 428 Mountain View Dr., Pahlonega, Georgia 30533. Call for phone # or just call information**. His father has pancreatic and liver cancer and was sent home to die. He had chemo and the cancer increased and he got sicker. He took aloe vera for 30 days and the tumor still increased. As he got sicker, his appetite got worse and he lost more weight. He is now eating just the seeds every day and has gained back his weight because his appetite returned. He is due for a CAT scan soon. He is still tired through the day. **(Note. Please remember to eat foods with B17 so you never have to deal with cancer.)**

22nd November 1997

I think it's possible that a combination of radiation and the Vitamin B17 completely disintegrates a tumor. This had happened with a few people already where the doctors said the radiation was only supposed to shrink it a little. Report today that **Jason McNally's (Call for phone #)** face tumor is completely gone after less than three weeks (taking Vitamin B17, seeds and 2 radiation treatments). He originally had lung cancer and no CAT scan has been taken that I am aware of showing his lung condition. He feels normal and drives a cab all day.

25th November 1997

Tabatha Dicus has just had a CAT scan and nodules in her lung were found. They were biopsied as cancer. She's already been through massive chemo and radiation for years and had started the seeds and vitamin about 5 months ago. For the last few months she's only been taking small amounts of B17. I believe that if your body already had cancer and you've been through chemo you need higher maintenance dosages after the first two months of high doses. She's started up again. (Update 4/6/98 she's doing fine just started a home business)

Sandy Williams reported today that her skin cancer has grown back after she stopped eating the seeds. When she took the seeds a couple of months ago the skin cancer went away (in a week or two). When she stopped it came back. She will now take some pictures, start the seeds again and then take some pictures when it goes away.

P.S. We need all of the pictures, reports and records and prayer we can get. An FDA agent was at my house last week for two hours as I gave him the info he wanted.

14th December 1997
Warren Tetting has been eating the seeds and his skin cancer has finally stopped growing back. He has had operations on his head where they tried to take the small cancer out by digging down to his skull and it always grew back. Write him if you want... much of his family has died from cancer. **1063 W. 7th St. Saint Pauls, MN. 55102.**

16th December 1997
Patricia Ritter called three weeks ago and said that she had a skin melanoma the size of a quarter. I told her to take pictures because in less than a couple of weeks it would be mostly gone if she eats the seeds. Today I talked with her and it has gone down more then 50% in size. She should saturate her body even more now. If you would like to know the progress of her condition, write her. Her mailing address is **5875 Knight Rd. Kingsley, MI 49649.**

12th January 1998
Spoke to **George Robinson** this weekend and his father who was terminal with lung cancer just got checked up after doing both chemo and the B17. His cancer has shrunk down over 75% and the doctors are at a loss of words. They say that it looks as if he's going to be fine. He needs to stop the chemo now or it will kill him. **(810)502-5055.**

24th January 1998
Patricia Ritter's skin melanoma (see 16/12) on her arm had incurred some strange reactions. After the melanoma shrunk down from the size of a quarter to the size of a pea it stayed the size of a pea for a couple of

days. She kept eating the seeds and then the pea-size tumor looked like it was opening up and caused her whole arm to swell. After about a week, the swelling went down and now even the pea-size tumor is gone.

John Yeber had the cancer in the jaw with incredible pain... he started the seeds and the B17 (supplement tablets) and the pain went away...he stopped the B17 and the pain came back. He started the B17 again and in a couple of days the pain went away again. **(305)580-5471**

Toby Cedarbaum (mentioned 11/17) called to say she now has absolutely no pain in her breast and the tumors are completely gone, except for some small calcium deposits.

29th January 1998
Today I have had more success phone calls than a hospital gets in a year. **Joseph Allen** has been suffering from cancer since the 70's. He has recently been tested with high counts in his blood indicating cancer. A mole (most likely cancerous) has begun to grow out of control for a month now. Immediately this mole has gone away within a week or so of being on the B17. **(713)473-4956**

Barb Cressman's husband had non-Hotchkins Lymphoma in the lining of his stomach. He started the B17 and seeds. Was just retested and 100% of the cancer cells are gone. He had an actual biopsy of the stomach. Her address is **Box 234, Crown, Saskatchewan, Canada.**

Jerry Butler's father was given a few weeks to live back in Sept. He has liver and pancreatic cancer. I spoke to him today and he told me that his father started taking the seeds back in September and immediately his appetite came back and I think he said that he gained weight. It's 5 months later and his father is fine. More energy, we're waiting for another scan. His phone # **(706)864-4781.**

Gino Cosentino called today to report about his aunt who had breast cancer that metastasized to her ribs and all throughout her liver. Her cancer had been constantly growing. She started the B17 and in two weeks her scan showed that it had stopped growing (it probably stopped the day she started the B17). Today is two months and her scan has shown that the cancer in the ribs is completely gone and the cancer in the liver is over half gone... she has been taking chemo all along as well as grape seed, Vitamin E, Essiac and Immunical. Chemo doesn't make cancer just go away, it might shrink it for a little while. Contact me for

188

Gino's number. He will tell you the story and give you his aunt's phone if needed. She has been taking about 2,000 mg of B17 per day and not many seeds.

14th February 1998

Lilian Morales has been treating two people. One lady has had bone cancer and tumors all along her spine for five years now. Her skin on her back is like chicken skin due to radiation burn. Her name is **Maria Gonzales** and she hasn't been able to drive for the last five years because of the pain...she has been in and out of chemo and radiation with no real difference in the pain or tumor sizes. She started the B17 and seeds a few months ago and the tumors have shrunk down and she is now driving again for the first time in five years... she claims she is doing 200% better...she has still been taking some chemo.

Lilian Morales' other patient, **Angelita Corrales** has diabetes and ovarian cancer. She started the seeds back in Sept. She has just done the seeds and no chemo or vitamin B17 (tablets). She had previously had a biopsy that showed ovarian cancer. She just had another test and the cancer is not there anymore. This is a common case. I have seen nothing but complete cancer disappearance in cervical and ovarian. I have not yet seen the B17 not work (excuse the grammar). **Lilian Morales'** phone # is **(915)821-5860**

Bart Bartholomew had small cell cancer in his lung and was given about 6 months to live with the chemo...this was about 4 months ago...he started the B17 and the seeds and also the chemo... The cancer has shrunk greatly. The doctors of course don't understand what's going on.... they think they're so successful they're going to give him full doses of radiation. ...I can't convince him to stop the radiation and that the remaining tissue is just scar tissue... radiation can only hurt him now... His phone is **(561)286-6115.**

18th March 1998

After months of giving the therapy to others we have our first results on bone cancer combined with chemotherapy. Chemotherapy alone might slow bone cancer down but in the end it cannot stop it. **Sally Barnette** has been taking the seeds and the B17 and took some chemo. She had bone cancer about 4 months ago. Her latest scan showed no bone cancer at all. Her address is 70 Lower Airport Road, Lumberton, Mississippi.

Billy Zombrewski - Here is a typical story. Billy and his wife have been taking the B17 and the seeds. Now they are just taking the seeds.

Both Billy and his wife have moles that have fallen off which they've had for years. Billy used to have back pain and body aches for years that all seemed to have gone away. Billy tossed and turned for 20 years as he slept and now his wife claims that he no longer does that. Billy says that he went to sleep the other night and actually woke up in the same position. (Woke up the next morning in the same position not 5 minutes later...haha) Who knows what was growing and going on in their bodies. These are just stories I get when I happen to ask someone who is reordering about their conditions. In other words, these are the tip of the iceberg. In the future we will have more organized studies and support groups. Billy's address is **9823 KINDLE TREE CIRCLE, Houston TX.77040**.

Mr Pavlov had intestinal cancer to the point that they opened him up to operate and then just shut him up again because the cancer was too far gone. They gave him chemo in the hope of shrinking it so that they could go in and operate at a later date. The day he started the chemo he started eating 5 seeds per hour religiously. Two months later they opened him up again to try to get the infesting cancer out. They closed him up and the report said "no recurring tumor". Do you see.... the report said no recurring tumor and the cancer was never taken out in the first place. I have this oncology report in my files and have read it myself. Mr. Pavlov's phone # is (718)497-1897. His intestinal cancer is no more. Mr. Pavlov is from Croatia.

We have just had results from someone with brain cancer and they have experienced 33% tumor reduction according to their most recent brain scan. The doctor is taking extensive notes about the seeds that **Mr. Herbert** is taking because he's never seen anything like this. The tumor part that is left in the brain is most probably scar tissue, according to the doctor. This goes with everyone when it comes to detecting if a tumor is scar tissue or real live tumor. THE MRI CANNOT TELL THE DIFFERENCE BETWEEN TUMOR, DEAD TUMOR AND SCAR TISSUE. Anyway **Mr. Herbert's address is 2 King Arthur, Boxford, Mass. 01921** and his phone # is **(978)887-0153**. Please only call him if you have a similar cancer.

This letter was received today from **Lee Tessina**
"I'm glad to see that someone has finally gotten this information onto the web. In 1980, at age 40, I was diagnosed with Hodgkin's, nodular scleroses(sp) stage one...After 4 months of staging, during which I did NOT allow any invasive surgery, other than a small biopsy on my neck at

190

the site of a swollen lymph gland, and a bone marrow test (very painful), I declined the offer of chemotherapy, declined the offer of radiation, and instead used B17, both by injection of laetrile, and by apricot kernels. I also changed my diet, and started taking MEGA doses of certain vitamins and minerals prescribed by a nutritionist. In 1990, I was told I was "cancer-free" by the same doctor who originally diagnosed me. I have had no further problems with cancer..."

4th April 1998

Ruth Helm is another that did the right thing. She was diagnosed with breast cancer and started the seeds right away... She called today and told me how her breast cancer shrunk down all the way with the seeds but was still on schedule for chemo. She received one session of chemo and the doctor couldn't in good conscience continue with the chemo...(not all doctors will do this) He told her she was cancer-free... She now continues with the seeds as every human should...phone # is **(724)495-2195**.

Judy Reesh has a dog that had a tumor in its mouth (cancerous). She crushed up seeds and put them in the dog's food for a while and the tumor went away.... Actually there's still a little lump but that's most definitely scar tissue and benign tumor... However, it shrunk down at least 90%. Call for her phone #.

I am hearing cases of people with liver and pancreas cancer who are taking the seeds and the cancer is shrinking all the way down to about 10 or 20 percent of what it was originally. At this point some people are under the wrong impression. They feel that the tumor is supposed to go away 100% and therefore go ahead with massive chemo. Good does not happen when they do this.

* * * * *

Donald Factor is the son of cosmetics entrepreneur Max Factor. Donald tells how B17 Metabolic Therapy in Doctor Contreras' Oasis of Hope Clinic saved his life. This November (1999), Donald is overjoyed to celebrate 13 years of further life (and still counting!) – life that orthodox medicine was unable to grant him:

My name is Donald Factor. I was living in London in November of 1986 when I was diagnosed with carcinoma of the lung that had spread to my liver. Basically the doctors in England didn't hold a lot of hope for me. They were very apologetic and offered a treatment which they thought might extend my life for a little while, but not for very long. I didn't feel like accepting that prognosis and decided to go and see Dr Contreras.

I'd met Dr Contreras a few years before in a conference in England and was very impressed with his approach. He told us they used modern medicine combined with other natural things and a lot of love and faith. My wife and I moved from England to Los Angeles and then we drove down to Tijuana to the Oasis hospital where I was treated.

When I arrived I was in an extremely weak condition. It was 10 days after the original diagnosis and the cancer had spread to my spine. I was in excruciating pain with my sciatic nerve affected so I could hardly walk. I was loosing weight rapidly too. They took a look at me at the Contreras clinic and were quite concerned. They too were not very optimistic about my future, but as Dr Contreras Sr. said, because both I and my wife were very committed to doing everything possible to beat the cancer, they were prepared to work with us.

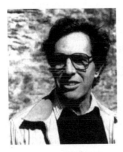

To make a long story short, the treatment succeeded. I knew Tijuana. I was born and raised in Los Angeles, and it was a place we used to go to do naughty things when we were teenagers. It wasn't ever a place that I associated with getting well, rather a place that I associated with getting sick.

I was very impressed with the Contreras clinic when I went inside and met the people; I had never experienced a hospital where the doctors would treat me as a human being instead of a bunch of symptoms or a disease walking through the door. Suddenly, there was a team of people there who were interested in me and they were involving me in the course my treatment would take. I was being asked, I was being informed and suddenly I was part of the team that was treating me. I wasn't just an object that was being treated. And that was tremendous and I realized there was another side to Tijuana that I never imagined possible in my youth.

This all happened in 1986 so it will be 13 years this November. After the initial metabolic treatment and about a year of home therapy, I was totally clear of any sign of cancer. I went back regularly for check-ups and after about three years of being in remission, the doctors said I was cured. I said, 'I thought in the cancer business you were never cured.' And they said, ' Well it is silly to keep writing down 'Remission' year after year. We'll see you whenever you want to come back.' And that was that.

I already had a lot of ideas about the orthodoxy, I suppose I'd call it, of modern science. I was never happy with it. I had known people with HIV and AIDS and I was always rather disturbed at the way that disease was treated and how in those days it seemed that anyone who was diagnosed with HIV was dead within a couple of years. It didn't seem right to me, it seemed to me that there was something else and I knew a bit about alternatives and complimentary medicine. My wife had been involved with some hands on healing work before that, so I was very open to other ways of doing things. I had never had a direct experience myself as a patient being involved in a place where love and human kindness were actually applied as part of the program. I have to say it was a revelation.

My name has been given to people and I have happily talked with them telling them pretty much what I tell you now. I think one of the main things that helped early on in my treatment was the use of a catheter which was able to feed the IV medications directly into my liver. I think it was a Hickman catheter inserted into my umbilical vein that was able to stay in for about a year. It made taking all the medication much easier. One could simply inject whatever was needed into the end of a plastic tube and it would get through the catheter to the body without the worry of needles and veins. That was wonderful. It made life much easier and the quality of the treatment better. It worked amazingly."

* * * * *

18th February 2000 (Non-Hodgkins Lymphoma)
Michael Roy knew that some type of lymphoma was forming in his body about 5 years ago. Upon diagnosis at the end of 1999, it was discovered that he had Non-Hodgkins Lymphoma small cell follicular. By December the tumours were getting painful and larger. On 24th December Michael started the apricot seeds and the B17, fresh pineapple, Vitamin C and one or two backup treatments. In two days the pain went away and the tumours began shrinking under his arm and on his neck. When he went to the oncologist, the latter said that the tumours under the arm were completely gone and the other had shrunk. On Michael's way home from the oncologist he wrecked his brand new car. He told the police officer at the scene (who happened to be a friend of his) "It just doesn't matter!!! I'm better from cancer," and continued to tell the officer his story. (e-mail Michael at aptoroy@yahoo.com)

19th February 2000 (Stage 4 lung cancer)
After years of routine visits to the doctors and getting a clean bill of health, **Stella Foster** was diagnosed with Stage 4 lung cancer with involvement in both lungs in July 1999. Following the advice of her doctor, Stella started chemotherapy immediately in an effort to 'control' her

condition.[183] After only one chemo treatment she was admitted to the hospital for five days with seizures and almost died. Early in December of 1999 she decided to try Metabolic Therapy with Vitamin B17 and added Essiac Tea to her therapy. After 2 1/2 months on Metabolic Therapy, her cancer had completely GONE.

On 9th February 2000 she showed up at the doctor's office to find out the status of her condition. She describes being afraid when the doctor walked in looking pale after reading her results. The doctor was pale and his mouth had dropped, not because she was sick, but because her lungs were completely clear of cancer. This is one of a growing number of cases establishment medicine calls 'spontaneous regression' or 'a miracle'.

7th March 2000 (Carcinoma of the lip)

Ann Harris was diagnosed with carcinoma of the lip in 1991 (9 years ago). The cancer never went away despite three surgeries and one session of radiation. The tumour was located on one side of her mouth and extended all the way into the mouth, causing so much pain that she could not eat. After starting Metabolic Therapy on 9th November 1999, within 10 days she saw that her tumour began to try up and shrink dramatically. She is now on her fourth month of Metabolic Therapy and says her tumour is almost gone.

Had Mrs Harris known about Vitamin B17 9 years ago, it would have saved her 9 years of pain and suffering.

3rd March 2000 (Squamous cell carcinoma)

On 3rd July 1999 **Mr Darrell Derusha** was diagnosed with squamous cell carcinoma. He had a big lump in his neck about the size of a plum and one in his throat which he could feel every time he swallowed. On 14th January 2000 Darrell decided to start Metabolic Therapy and Metabolic Therapy only to correct his condition. After only one month the tumour in the neck was reduced to the size of a marble (from resembling a plum). One day he felt something bothering his throat and proceeded to cough. Much to his amazement the tumour he had in his throat came out and he describes it as follows: "It was about the size of a grape and it was dead, dry, and had some blood on it." Ever since, Mr Derusha has not felt the bother inside his throat. He is now feeling great and continues on his way to recovery.

---

[183] Eight out of every ten patients with cancer of the lung, who choose to submit to orthodox therapy, will be dead within one year. Ninety-five out of every one hundred patients with cancer of the lung will be dead five years following diagnosis if they choose only orthodox therapy. (*Clinical Oncology for Medical Students and Physicians*, op. cit., p. 99.)

Date: Tue, 12 Oct 1999 15:54:05 +0100
From: "Tony Wakefield" - tony.wakefield@virgin.net
To: "David Arjona" dearjona@idt.net (World Without Cancer, Inc)

Dear David
I have recently started taking B17 in seed form following my recent order, following completion of Phase I & 2 Metabolic Therapy with oral B-17. Recently had good test results showing that my bladder cancer is in remission and that I only have a very small area of low-grade cancer in my prostrate which was almost undetectable.

Is the seed form sufficient for ongoing treatment or should I revert to the Metabolic Therapy? I am taking at the moment the recommended 1 seed for every 10 pounds of body weight.

I know you are not a doctor and I hope you do not mind the question - I do not have anyone in the UK who I can ask the question.

Regards

Tony Wakefield,
232 High Road,
Byfleet, Surrey,
KT14 7DD, England

The following e-mail was received by retired Royal Navy Commander Geoff Sherman from a member of his e-mailing list. Geoff and Phillip Day often share B17/amygdalin updates for dissemination and use media like the Internet to reach as many people as possible.

To: GJTSherman@aol.com <GJTSherman@aol.com>
28th September 1999
Dear Geoff
I thought you would like to know about my father-in-law who was diagnosed with Hodgkin's Disease last year (which is cancer of the lymph system) - he had been very run down for a long period of time having to cope with my mother-in-law who had been getting progressively worse with Alzheimer's.
He got so run down and weary with life that his immune system just collapsed and he got these nodules growing at the base side of his neck. He eventually resorted to go to Christie's in Manchester for radiotherapy

and he lost half the hair on one side of his head, apart from feeling dreadful.

Following the six-week course the specialist said that it looked as though they had caught the cancer in time before it started to spread through the rest of his lymphatic system - he was very relieved.

Several weeks later - guess what - the nodules started growing again - my father in law certainly did not want to have radiation again and resigned himself to the fact that the cancer was going to kill him and there was nothing that he could do about it.

Just at that time you had started to e-mail me with info about Vitamin B17 and I decided to order it for my father in law. I gave him a bag of apricot kernels and a tub of 500mg B17 tablets - which he took religiously until he had finished them. He felt quite ill and sick when he was on them, but the nodules started to shrink after three weeks. On visiting the specialist several weeks later, the specialist could not believe that the most recent scan showed no sign of the cancer - he was truly amazed and asked my father in law to return again 6 weeks later - just to make sure.

After 6 weeks and a further scan the specialist confirmed his earlier statement that the cancer has indeed gone! - he does not want to see my father in law now for a further 6 months! - Everyone is very happy again now - all thanks to B17.

All thanks and praise to you, Geoff, for helping to spread the life-saving word!

David Thompson

From: gradym@kdi.com (**Janice Manley**)
Hi...

"Well, this was the basis of the Laetrelle (sp?) cancer regimen that my mother did in the 60s. She was given 6 months to live and started on standard chemotherapy. Each treatment was to last 5 days, then 5 days of being sick and 20 days of "normal" life. She was sick 30 days (vomiting, diahhh (sp???)). After 4 months, she said she'd rather be dead, but instead she went to Mexico and did Laetrelle...got pills that were made of seed pits....she ate lots of apricot pits because that was supposed to be the best. So... I guess if you look at her, she's a 100% testimony. Given 6 months to live, she lived 20 more years after she did the pit business."

Edward Rudolph had colon and lung cancer and prostate cancer. He started the vitamin B17 (500 mg. tablets) and the seeds about a month ago. He was in pain in his lungs and his colon. There was a tumor in his lower intestinal area that was the size of an egg which could be felt. The

196

tumor, in 30 days is now hardly detectable and the pain is no more. His phone # is (313)942-1026. His e-mail address is earjlm@earth*%*.com.

Testimonials from G Edward Griffin's *World Without Cancer*

Mr David Edmunds of Pinole, California, was operated on in June of 1971 for cancer of the colon, which also had metastasized or spread to the bladder. When the surgeon opened him up, he found that the malignant tissue was so widespread it was almost impossible to remove it all. The blockage of the intestines was relieved by severing the colon and bringing the open end to the outside of his abdomen -- a procedure known as Colonostomy. Five months later, the cancer had worsened, and Mr. Edmunds was told that he had only a few more months to live.

Mr. Edmunds, who is a registered nurse, had heard about laetrile and decided to give it a try. Six months later, instead of lying on his deathbed, Mr. Edmunds surprised his doctors by feeling well enough to resume an almost normal routine. An exploratory cystoscopy of the bladder revealed that the cancer had disappeared. At his own insistence, he was admitted to the hospital to see if his colon could be put back together again. In surgery, they found nothing even resembling cancer tissue. So they reconnected the colon and sent him home to recuperate. It was the first time in the history of the hospital that a *reverse* colostomy for this condition had been performed. At the time of the author's last contact three years later, Mr. Edmunds was living a normal life of health and vigor.

In Walnut Creek, California, **Mrs. Joanne Wilkinson**, mother of six, had a tumor removed from her left leg just below the thigh. Four months later there was a recurrence requiring additional surgery and the removal of muscle and bone. A year later, a painful lump in the groin appeared and began to drain. A biopsy revealed that her cancer had returned and was spreading. Her doctor told her that surgery would be necessary again, but this time they would have to amputate her leg at the hip, and probably the bladder and one of the kidneys as well. The plan was to open up her lungs first to see if cancer had located there. If it had, then they would not amputate, because there would be no chance of saving her anyway.

At the urging of her sister and of a mutual friend, Mrs. Wilkinson decided not to undergo surgery but to try laetrile instead. Her doctor was greatly upset by this and told her that, if she did not have the surgery, she couldn't possibly live longer than twelve weeks. Mrs. Wilkinson describes in her own words:

"I will never forget that day! It was a Saturday and the stitches from the biopsy were still in the leg. Dr Krebs gave me an injection of laetrile and the tumor reacted. It got very large -- from walnut size to the size of a small lemon -- and there was bleeding for four or five days. I went back on

Monday, Wednesday and Friday each week for five weeks to get injections, and the tumor then started getting smaller. Five weeks later I could no longer feel it. An X-ray was taken the first Monday, and regularly after that to watch the progress. Injections were continued for six months -- 10 cc's three times a week and of course the diet: No dairy products, nothing made with white flour, -- no eggs --but white fish, chicken, turkey.

I felt wonderful, and in fact, 9 months later, the doctor told me I needed no more injections. My X-rays were clear, showing that the tumor had shrunk, was apparently encased in scar tissue, and was not active."

The author's last contact with Mrs. Wilkinson was nine years later after her doctor told her she couldn't possibly live longer than twelve weeks without surgery. She was living a healthy and productive life, and all that was left as a grim reminder of her narrow escape was a small scar from the biopsy.

Mr. **Joe Botelho** of San Pablo, California, underwent surgery (trans-urethral resection) and was told by his doctor that he had a prostate tumor that simply had to come out. His reaction?

"I didn't let them take it out because I figured that would only spread it. The doctor told me I wouldn't last too long. He wanted to give me cobalt, and I wouldn't agree to that either. At a health food store I heard about a doctor in San Francisco who used laetrile. I went to see him, was told that the prostate was the size of a bar of soap. I got one injection every four days for several months."

Mr. Botelho, who was sixty five at the time, also maintained a strict diet designed specifically not to use up the body's pancreatic enzyme, trypsin. When the author interviewed him three years later, his tumor was gone, and he even reported that his hair was turning dark again. He was not sure what was causing that, but attributed it to his better eating habits.

Alicia Buttons, the wife of the famous actor-comedian Red Buttons, is among the thousands of Americans who attribute their lives to the action of laetrile. Speaking before a cancer convention in Los Angeles, Red Buttons declared:

"Laetrile saved Alicia from cancer. Doctors here in the U.S. gave her only a few months to live last November. But now she is alive and well, a beautiful and vital wife and mother, thanks to God and to those wonderful men who have the courage to stand up for their science."

Mrs. Buttons had been suffering from advanced cancer of the throat and was given up as terminal by practitioners of orthodox medicine. As a last resort, however, she went to West Germany to seek laetrile therapy from Dr Hans Nieper of the Silbersee Hospital in Hanover. Within a few months her cancer had completely regressed, the pain had gone, her appetite had returned, and she was as healthy and strong as ever. Doctors in the United States verified the amazing recovery, but could not believe that a mere vitamin substance had been responsible. Alicia is still going strong twenty-three years later.

The following letter from **Bud Robinson** in Phoenix, Arizona, needs no further comment. It was sent to Dr Ernest Krebs Jr.

Dear Dr Krebs,
Thank you for giving me another birthday (May 17). Please, again, remember November 15, 1979, when my doctor and four other urologists gave me a maximum of four months to live with my prostate cancer, and they set up appointments for radiation and chemotherapy, which I knew would kill me if the cancer didn't, and refused their treatment.
Then on a Sunday afternoon I contacted you by telephone and went with your simple program.
I am 71 years old and am on my 13th year [of survival]. Three of the four urologists have died with prostate cancer, and forty or fifty people are alive today, and doing well, because they followed my "Krebs" simple program.
Thanks again for giving me back my life.
Your friend,
HM "Bud" Robinson

This letter was written in 1992. When the Mr Griffin contacted him in June of 1996, Mr. Robinson was still going strong and the number of cancer patients he had helped to recover was up to 90.

Dec. 27th 1998

Dear Jason

I have a patient (39 yr old female) who had a 3 1/2cm malignant breast tumor that continued to regrow after three separate chemo cycles in the past 2 years. She was also on Tamoxifen daily and had radiation treatments. She was tired of dealing with the side effects and lack of results and was referred to my office. She was on 20-30 seeds and about 3,000mg of B17 per day for less than 3 weeks before going back to her oncologist. They told her they wanted to remove her breast and follow up with more chemo and she refused. They retested her that day and the results showed that the tumor shrank to 1/2cm and was no longer malignant.

Another patient (30 yr old female) came into the office with a 6cm brain tumor in late September. Over the summer she had surgery to remove a tumor and it grew back in less than 3 months. She was on chemo when she came in and we put her on 45 seeds a day as well as some supplements to support her adrenals and thymus gland. Also a complete digestive enzyme complex was added. She had another MRI done on 12-10-98 and the tumor shrunk to about 1 1/2cm and the neuro-oncologist thinks the remainder of the tumor is just scar tissue. Now he wants to know what she has been doing and also stated that he doesn't believe radiation helps with brain tumors. She is preparing a full testimony for us and will send it along. Thank you for your efforts in getting out the seeds and the truth!!

I also have a patient whose dog was lame in his back legs and none of the top vets in the area had any hope for him. Two seeds a day and he is running around like a puppy. I will try for a testimony on him too. Let me know the latest with the FDA, they scare me but I know the Lord will protect us. Hope you had a blessed Christmas.

Yours in good health,
Thomas Von Ohlen, M.S.
Clinical Nutritionist

Advanced Center For Nutrition
336 Round Hill Road
Fairfield CT 06430 (203)319-1274

TESTIMONIES FROM NEWAYS CUSTOMERS

Ever since I was little, I had been blessed with good health. Consequently I took my health for granted – that is, until the age of 38 when my life was turned upside down. I was diagnosed with fibromyalgia and chronic fatigue syndrome. My body developed 30 other symptoms over a two-year span that complicated my health. I had been an active person all my life with strong athletic interests, but now I lived in chronic pain 24 hours a day. At one point my illness was so overwhelming I could no longer do the simple tasks required in my daily routine. I was treated with anti-inflammatory and anti-depressant drugs, but the side-effects were so strong that I was switched every three weeks to counter the effects. I was placed on uppers and downers at the same time to keep me alive from day to day. As I was pulled off the drugs, I was later placed on an addicting drug without my knowledge. I was told that I'd be on drugs and live in pain for the rest of my life.

Then through the grace of God, I found an acupuncturist who introduced me to the concept of potentially cancer-causing agents in personal care products. After checking my bathroom, I was amazed at the number of expensive products I owned containing toxic ingredients. I could no longer justify using these products and converted my bathroom products over immediately to the alternatives manufactured by Neways International. I started using their anti-ageing nutritional products, and within a few months my health improved in minute stages. After a 2-year commitment of using carcinogen-free products, I have regained my total health. **Billie Jo Fiege. Menomonie, WI, USA**

Hello. My name is Ardie Friend. I worked for a major cosmetics company and contracted chemical poisoning after years of showing and telling their products and fragrances. I was bedridden, could only go from my bed to the couch and barely had the strength even to take a shower. My husband had to take over all the household responsibilities. When he wasn't there, I felt so ill, I didn't even have the energy to cook my food, so I ate it cold and then went back to bed.

I learned about harmful ingredients in common household products from a radio show in Youngstown, Ohio. After checking all the labels of my own cosmetic products (which naturally I had obtained through my employers), I realized I could never return to work. After a doctor formally diagnosed me with chemical poisoning, I immediately threw all those products in the garbage and purchased the harmless alternatives provided by Neways International. After a while, I began to feel better. I remember my doctor saying that if ever I returned to work and continued the poisoning of my body, he may not be able to bring me back a second time. I was taking Neways' Revenol and later added their nutritional product Maximol. While I was taking these products, it was weird – I could actually feel my body and head clearing and the strength flowing back.

I used to have headaches, nausea, migraines, vomiting and diarrhea on a daily basis. All these symptoms disappeared when I commenced taking the Maximol. They have never returned in 3 years.

My husband Norman would also like to tell you about our son Scott.

Norman: Our son Scott has also had a dramatic experience with chemical poisoning. During the Gulf War, Scott was stationed on the front line as a mechanic working on Cobra attack helicopters. The area was close to the oil fires that were burning out of control in the Kuwaiti desert. When he returned to the United States after the war, his health rapidly deteriorated to where he was skin and bones, had dark circles under his eyes and was chronically fatigued. One night when our son visited us for dinner, he was so emaciated that we asked him outright if he was doing drugs. He responded that since he had returned home, he was so sick, he would go 2-3 days without sleep, he was having hallucinations and didn't know what to do about his health.

We took him to the Veteran's Administration (VA) hospital in Canton, Ohio, but they said there was nothing wrong with him. Later we went to a world-famous clinic in Cleveland and they studied my son. They also said there was nothing wrong, but gave him a prescription which they said would make him forget anything he thought was wrong with him. Scott gave the drugs back after he saw the word 'Prozac' on the prescription. He told them he already had enough chemicals in his body. It was strange but we were never billed for that particular consultation.

We knew that many veterans were returning from the war in Kuwait with health problems, so a short time later, we found a doctor who was qualified to run certain tests on my son. He found that Scott had been poisoned with military-grade anthrax and mustard gas. Other caustic chemicals were also found in his blood. Scott began building his system up with the antioxidant compound Revenol and other products from Neways, such as Maximol, Ming Gold and Emperor's Formula. He also started on the product Purge, which is a parasite cleanser.

After only a few days, to our distress, things got pretty dramatic: a bulge appeared on Scott's temple the size of a golf ball which began to drain foul liquids. All along the top of his collarbone, an awful lesion appeared that looked like a raised blood-blister. In the middle of his chest another golf-ball-sized lump appeared which was hard. He stuck it with a straight pin but only managed to bend the pin. When he pulled the pin out, all this foul stuff oozed out, rank in smell. All along his hairline, a series of angry, oil-like blackheads appeared. All over the top of his head, marks appeared that looked like someone had punctured his scalp with pins. He had breakouts all over his body, including another lump on the side of his mouth under the jawbone. Another appeared on his cheekbone. This was a man who used to be a model. It was heartbreaking for him and us to see our healthy boy go from total health to someone who looked like they has been locked up in a concentration camp.

But we all knew the bad stuff was leaving. Scott continued with the Neways products and today has 90% of his health back. Every six months, our son does a round of Neways' Purge to continue ridding himself of the chemical poisoning he received in the Persian Gulf War. We're just so happy to have our precious son back with us and well once more. We all know now how close we came to losing him.
Norman and Ardie Friend
nfriend@gateway.net

My name is Lynae Jorgenson. I began hairdressing at the age of 15. When I was 24, I began suffering from a host of degenerative illnesses. I was diagnosed with pelvic inflammatory disease and had a partial hysterectomy. My first child was born when I was 27 years old. Shortly after his birth, I began having problems that required D&Cs. During my second pregnancy, I threatened to miscarry during the 6th month. I was finally able to go to term but after delivery had four more D&Cs. When I was 36 years old, I ended up with a complete hysterectomy.

Shortly after, I was diagnosed with osteoarthritis. Within four years I had four knee surgeries. At age 41, I had my first hip replaced due to total disintegration of the hip joint. By my 14th year of marriage, I had undergone 15 surgeries. In 1998, I had my other hip replaced because of its total disintegration. The pain I was now suffering was excruciating. I was still trying maintain a normal work schedule but my deteriorating condition soon got the better of me and I began to spend more and more time in bed.

Shortly before my second hip replacement in January 1998, I heard a woman talking about toxins and what they do to our bodies. I realized immediately that the stories she was telling about people and what chemicals can do to their bodies related to me. You see, even though the doctors were diagnosing me with osteoarthritis, they were consistently failing to find a 'sed' rate – a blood indicator signifying arthritis.

My second hip replacement operation was a nightmare. My recovery was so slow and erratic that my doctors became concerned whether I would ever get out of the wheelchair again. At that time I was in a full body brace, even though I had only had hip surgery.

It was shortly after this surgery that I started reading a book I had picked up from the woman who was speaking about toxic ingredients. As I read, I realized that my problem was probably toxicity and that I had been poisoned by the chemicals I'd been using for years in hairdressing. Blood analysis indicated that my liver had been severely damaged. I was told there were only three chemicals that could cause liver damage to this degree. One of those was sodium lauryl sulfate, one of the main ingredients in the shampoos I had been using for years.

For the previous 28 years, I had performed between 10 and 12 shampoos a day, which is probably why I had such a complete body breakdown at an early age. I knew that I could never return to my profession so I began investigating other alternatives. At this time I was introduced to Neways International and began taking their nutritional supplements on a daily basis, as well as replacing my toxic household and personal care products. It was after 5 months of taking these supplements, doing whatever exercise I could do, and the help and faith of my family, that my health improved.

I used to wake up wishing my life would end. Now I wake up full of energy and vigor for the day. I believe to this day that the Neways supplements quite literally saved my life.
Lynae Jorgenson, Burnsville, MN, USA

My name is Joe Hornsey. I am what one would describe as the ultimate Type A behavioral person. Having been the CEO of five different corporations during my career, a member of practically every business committee in town and a candidate for the Texas Congress, I felt that I could burn the candle at both ends. After all, heart attacks happen to other people.

At the age of 37 I had my first heart attack. Nine years later I had my second attack but this time the doctors had to do by-pass surgery for seven clogged arteries. Even though I had made some lifestyle and diet changes, I still had the second heart attack, this time doing damage to my heart.

Eleven years later I felt that I was clogging up again, so I went to see one of the top cardiologists in San Antonio. After several tests he began to suggest surgery again. At this point in my life I had begun to learn more about alternative healthcare and had been introduced to Neways International in Salem, Utah. So I asked the doctor about chelation treatments as an alternative to open heart surgery. What I got in return was a twenty-minute lecture about quackery.

Since part of my college degree from Texas A&M University is in biochemistry and nutrition, I felt the idea of intravenous and oral chelation made too much sense to ignore. So I opted for chelation instead of surgery.

On 9th November 1998 my life changed. During that frightful night I experienced my third major heart attack. Although I did not go to the hospital until later the next day, what happened next was astounding. First, my enzyme count was so high the doctors felt two things should have happened: (1) I should not have lived and (2) if I did live, the damage to my heart should have been significant. Fortunately, neither of these things happened. My cardiologist could not believe it. The doctor who did my angioplasty said I had the best arteries he had ever seen. And to top it off, they found that my heart was growing a large number of collateral arteries. Reluctantly, my cardiologist admitted that the only reason that I'm alive today (15 months later) is that the products I had been taking during that two-year period had strengthened my heart and my arteries. Basically they saved my life and prevented additional damage to my heart. I can recommend without hesitation the nutritional value of Neways products --- specifically Maximol, Revenol, Orachel and Cardiol.
Joe Hornsey San Antonio, TX, USA

My name is Ivy Johnson III. I was involved in a serious motorcycle accident in 1986. I was unable to walk for two years. As a result of all the surgeries I was unable to work and was on the verge of bankruptcy. Over the course of the year, as a result of all the surgeries, I had three blood clots in my lungs. The only way I could consume food was in the prone position. As a result I developed a hiatus hernia and gained over 150lbs. After eight surgeries, I still could not stand on my legs without them filling up with water and blood (edema) and ultimately swelling larger than my hips.

They had rebuilt my left knee as a result of my ligaments being torn. I was a physical wreck. I was on powerful drugs to stop my body from producing stomach acid to prevent acid reflux, symptoms, which are indicative of a hiatus hernia. I was consuming enormous amounts of over-the-counter antacids to try and neutralize the stomach acids. I could feel a numbness in my chest and I was frightened that I was suffering a heart attack. Seventeen times in that year I was admitted to the emergency room at a local hospital because I felt I was dying. My parents recommended that I try the Neways supplements Revenol, Maximol and Youthinol. After one month I realized that I had not used my prescriptive and over-the-counter medications for over 30 days. Immediately the attack-like symptoms went from once a day to once a month. After four years with just the Neways nutritional supplements and with no additional surgeries, I can now stand on my feet for six to seven hours a day with no challenge. Revenol, Maximol, Ming Gold, Orachel, and Biogevity have saved my life. I literally cannot live without these products.
Ivy Johnson III, Atlanta, GA, USA

Contacts! Contacts! Contacts!

Neways International

...supplies a fabulous range of personal and household care items, free of suspected carcinogens and harmful compounds. These include extremely high quality cosmetics, shampoos, a complete bathroom change-out kit and many other day-to-day products. **Neways** also fields a complete stable of excellent nutritional support products such as Maximol, (Cascading) Revenol, Purge, Hawaiian Noni and Cassie-Tea. These products go through extra cleaning processes to ensure their quality and purity. A full range of product details and a comprehensive online store are available through the contacts below.

For More Information on How to Obtain Safe Personal Care Products, Apricot Kernels, B17 Metabolic Therapy Products or Extra Copies of This Book, Contact:

US Auto Orders: (309) 416 8714
UK Orders: (01622) 832386
USA, call 011 44 1622 832386
UK Fax: (0870) 137 7441
US Fax: (309) 416 8714
www.credence.org
e-mail: sales@credence.org

Check out our great web-site at www.credence.org for additional information, testimonies and an online book store. Buy copies of this book and others to send to all your friends and relatives. Or have us send them a free information pack. Maybe you know and love someone who is suffering from cancer but feel you cannot approach them directly because 'you are not a doctor'. Pop a book in an envelope and send them a copy anonymously! **Who do you know alive today who couldn't benefit from the information contained in this book?**

Book prices are discounted for volume and are available in the following packs: 1 book, 10 books, 25 books, 50 books and 100 books. Call for price details or see our web-site.

Health Review and Free Information Pack
What other book entitles you to a free magazine subscription and regular e-mail updates completely free? If you have not received these and have purchased this book, contact us immediately!

Credence Publications also sends hundreds of free information packs throughout the world every month to those who have requested them either for themselves or for interested friends and relatives. Those who receive such packs will receive our seasonal magazine *Health Review*, informing the reader of the latest developments on this exciting subject. If you would like to take advantage of this service, please supply the relevant mailing address details to our head office address below:

Credence Publications
PO Box 3
TONBRIDGE
Kent TN12 9ZY
England
infopack@credence.org

EClub Bulletins
On the 1st and 15th of each month, Credence sends out the EClub Internet bulletin to thousands of subscribers worldwide. This highly informative e-mail newsletter is available FREE to customers who have purchased this book or who have requested EClub. This terrific online bulletin contains the latest news and research on cancer and other vital health topics. DO NOT BE WITHOUT THIS GREAT RESOURCE! If you wish to subscribe, e-mail Credence EClub at eclub@credence.org with your free request.

Doctor Referrals
If you would like to speak to a qualified doctor with the view to commencing nutritional therapy for cancer, call Credence on

(01622) 832386 (from the UK) or 011 44 1622 832386 (from the US) and we will put you in touch with a professional who can give you further details.

The Cancer Prevention Coalition
Dr Samuel Epstein's highly recommended organisation and its mission can be viewed over the Internet. Dr Epstein discusses the failure of conventional treatments to halt the major cancers, as well as graphically highlighting the many conflicts of interest that exist globally between the chemical and medical industries. His reports are also online. **www.preventcancer.com**

And God said, "See I have given you every herb that yields seed which is on the face of the earth, and every tree whose fruit yields seed; <u>to you it shall be for food.</u> Also to every beast of the earth, to every bird of the air, and to everything that creeps on the earth, in which there is life, I have given every green herb for food." And it was so. (Gen 1:29-30)

(God speaks) **Also take for yourself wheat, barley, beans, lentils, millet and spelt; put them into one vessel, and make bread of them for yourself..."** (Eze 4:9)

"I am the Lord that heals you." (Exo 15:26)

(God speaks) **"My people perish through lack of knowledge."** (Hosea 4:6)

(God speaks) **"If you diligently heed the voice of the Lord your God and do what is right in His sight, give ear to His commandments and keep all His statutes, I will put none of the diseases on you which I have brought on the Egyptians."** (Exodus 15:26)

"There is nothing covered that will not be revealed, nor hidden that will not be known. Therefore whatever you have heard spoken in the dark will be heard in the light, and whatever you have spoken in the ear in inner rooms will be proclaimed on the housetops." (Luke 12:2-3)

God has chosen the foolish things of the world to confound the wise, and God has chosen the weak things of the world to confound the things which are mighty. (1 Cor 1:27)

Bibliography

WRITTEN REFERENCES

Allen, Isobel *Doctors and their Careers: A New Generation*, London: Policies Studies Institute, 1988 117
Amundsen, Roald *The Northwest Passage*, London and New York, 1908 73
Berglas, Alexander Preface to *Cancer: Nature, Cause and Cure*, Paris, 1957 72
Brand, Dr Paul *The Forever Feast*, Monarch Publications 1994 . 69
British Medical Journal 116, 118
Brown, Wood & Smith *Sodium Cyanide as a Cancer Chemotherapeutic Agent... Laboratory and Clinical Studies*, American Journal Obst. & Gynec., 80:907, 1960 106
Cancer News Journal 61
Christian Brothers, http://www.christianbrothers.com.................
.... 14, 17, 18, 19
Coop & Blakely *New Zealand Journal of Science & technology*, 28th February 1949 105
d'Raye, Tonita, *The Facts About Fluoride*, PO Box 21075, Keizer, OR 97307 USA 96
Day, Phillip & Steven Ransom *Exposing AIDS*, Credence Publications, 2000 .... 30, 67, 70
Day, Phillip *Plastic Smiles and Buried Files*, a special report. Credence Publications, 1999 70
DeMeo, James *Anti-Constitutional Activities and Abuse of Police Power*, http://id.mind.net/community/orgonelab/fda.htm. 63
Diamond, Dr John and Dr Lee Cowden *Alternative Medicine: The Definitive Guide to Cancer*, Future Medicine Publishing, Inc, 21-1/2 Main St, Tiburon, CA 94920... 21, 48
Diamond, Harvey & Marilyn *Fit For Life – Parts 1 & 2*, Little, Brown & Company, 1987 80
Economic Botany 23
Environment and Health News, Vol. 3, Jan 1998 20
Epstein, Samuel MD and David Steinman The Breast Cancer Prevention Program, Macmillan, USA, 1997 ISBN 0025361929 7
Franklin & Reid *Australian Veterinary Journal*, 100:92, 1944 ... 105

Index

Environmental Protection Agency (EPA), 82, 83, 84, 85, 86
Eskimaux, 71
Estrogen, 24
Ethoxylation, 93, 100

Trophoblast, 24

U

U S Congress, 39, 61
University of California at Berkeley (UCB), 23, 49
University of Illinois, 23
Urine, 25, 27
US Postal Service, 63

V

Vitamin B1, 36, 109, 128, 129, 131, 132, 134, 135, 136, 137
Vitamin B12, 131, 132

Vitamin B17, 23, 24, 25, 26, 36, 38, 42, 48, 49, 50, 51, 52, 56, 104, 105, 106, 109, 128, 129, 131, 132, 134, 135, 136, 137, 138
Vitamin B2, 135
Vitamin C, 30, 62, 130, 132, 136
Vitamin E, 136

W

Washington, President George, 120
Wilson, Dr Benjamin, 39